Praise for
Yoga as Embodied Resistance

"Anjali Rao's *Yoga as Embodied Resistance* is like a map to the hidden terrain of yoga's history. She offers us an eagle-eye view that lifts us above the clouds so we can see the rolling hills and endless ocean of yoga as it stretches far back in time and into the distant future. This perspective is a gift beyond measure, and I'm so grateful to Anjali for taking the time to do the research and reflection that is so needed.

As I traveled through this book, I not only found a way through the dark passages of yoga's history, I also had the privilege of meeting some incredible—and long-forgotten—figures who have helped to make yoga the powerful and transformational practice it is. I feel like this book is like a map back to the heart of yoga. A map that always leads me back to myself."

—JIVANA HEYMAN, author and founder of Accessible Yoga

"Anjali Rao's *Yoga as Embodied Resistance* introduces us to four often-overlooked feminist icons whose very presence troubles mainstream narratives. Rao's storytelling weaves the deeper meaning and history of yogic tradition with important corrections. We learn that transcending the self also means actively challenging social hierarchies. That spiritual devotion can be an experience of embodied pleasure or radical expression. That practice, like reality itself, always demands a play of sameness and difference, synthesis and identity."

—DR. ANYA FOXEN, associate professor at California Polytechnic State University

"*Yoga as Embodied Resistance* is a book I have long awaited. It conducts an exploratory historical analysis of yoga that contextualizes yoga's cultural power over the modern world, providing an important component in understanding the true layers of both what yoga has meant and what it *can* mean for us in the future. This ancient Vedic teaching has the power to transform us into being. It is a revolutionary tool, and Rao deftly takes us through its layers of history and resistance.

In times of such dissonance, people need connection to the power of radical thought, ancient teaching, and wisdom. This book is a template for self-actualization, asking important questions about who we are and where we can go collectively."

—FARIHA RÓISÍN, author of *Who Is Wellness For?*

"Let the unlearning begin. Anjali provides a brilliant intersection where all practitioners of yoga can meet and evolve."

—KATHRYN BUDIG, founder of Haus of Phoenix

"*Yoga as Embodied Resistance* offers a critical analysis of how we cannot separate practice from history or the current context. It calls attention to the sordid history of yoga and begs us not to believe we can transcend that history or how it ties to the current social, political, and cultural context. Rao acknowledges the need for us to contextualize the patterns of oppression that continue to replicate themselves within yoga and beyond. This book calls us into deeper awareness and action, and it will disrupt, in the best way, how we think of and practice yoga."

—MICHELLE CASSANDRA JOHNSON, author of *Skill in Action*, *Finding Refuge*, and *We Heal Together*

"Fierce voices like Anjali Rao's show us what's possible when writers are courageous enough to contend with yoga's entangled origins in Hindu and caste-based oppression while simultaneously politicizing its potential toward embodied resistance. Like the metaphorical quilt she references, Rao's text weaves critical analysis of historic texts, compelling storytelling, and reflective narrative toward a dismantling of neoliberal and Hindutva control over yoga's transnational circulation. May more yogis read it and politicize their practice toward interconnected freedom!"

—SHEENA SOOD, PhD, assistant professor of sociology at Delaware Valley University

"Anjali provides an intricate landscape of stories, complex history, and invitations to challenge one's assumptions in her book. Her evocative writing brings layers of emotions to the surface for me as I continue to explore my own relationship to yoga, my lineages, and what it means to be a steward of these practices. I've been waiting a long time to have a trusted resource on the history of yoga and resistance, one that is far from simple and pushes modern day approaches to yoga into necessary examination."

—MELISSA SHAH, yoga therapist

YOGA AS EMBODIED RESISTANCE

A Feminist Lens on Caste, Gender,
and Sacred Resilience in Yoga History

ANJALI RAO

FOREWORD BY
THENMOZHI SOUNDARARAJAN

North Atlantic Books
Huichin, unceded Ohlone land
Berkeley, California

North Atlantic Books
Huichin, unceded Ohlone land
2526 Martin Luther King Jr Way
Berkeley, CA 94704 USA
www.northatlanticbooks.com

Cover art of Radha and Krishna on a lotus flower courtesy of Raw Pixel under Creative Commons, flame © AlexeyPushkin via Getty Images.
Cover design by Jess Morphew
Book design by Happenstance Type-O-Rama

Printed in the United States of America

Yoga as Embodied Resistance: A Feminist Lens on Caste, Gender, and Sacred Resilience in Yoga History is sponsored and published by North Atlantic Books, an educational nonprofit that collaborates with partners to develop cross-cultural perspectives; nurture holistic views of art, science, the humanities, and healing; and seed personal and global transformation by publishing work on the relationship of body, spirit, and nature.

North Atlantic Books's publications are distributed to the US trade and internationally by Penguin Random House Publisher Services. For further information, visit our website at www.northatlanticbooks.com.

The authorized representative in the EU for product safety and compliance is Eucomply OÜ, Pärnu mnt 139b-14, 11317 Tallinn, Estonia, hello@eucompliancepartner.com, +33757690241.

Library of Congress Cataloging-in-Publication Data
Names: Rao, Anjali author
Title: Yoga as embodied resistance : a feminist lens on caste, gender, and
    sacred resilience in yoga history / Anjali Rao ; foreword by Thenmozhi
    Soundararajan.
Description: Huichin, unceded Ohlone land, Berkeley, California : North
    Atlantic Books, [2025] | Includes bibliographical references and index.
    | Summary: "Discusses the relationships between caste and gender in
    yoga"-- Provided by publisher.
Identifiers: LCCN 2025016529 (print) | LCCN 2025016530 (ebook) | ISBN
    9798889842774 trade paperback | ISBN 9798889842781 ebook
Subjects: LCSH: Yoga--History | Caste--Religious aspects--Hinduism | Gender
    identity--Religious aspects--Hinduism
Classification: LCC B132.Y6 R3568 2025 (print) | LCC B132.Y6 (ebook) |
    DDC 181/.4509--dc23/eng/20250530
LC record available at https://lccn.loc.gov/2025016529
LC ebook record available at https://lccn.loc.gov/2025016530

1 2 3 4 5 6 7 8 9 KPC 30 29 28 27 26 25

Contents

Foreword by Thenmozhi Soundararajan vii

Introduction 1

1 Origins of Yoga and Hinduism 23

2 Is Yoga Hindu? 47

3 Sulabha, the Rebellious Philosopher 79

4 The Dance of Radha 111

5 The Naked Truth Tellers 137

6 The Song of Piro .151

Conclusion: Embodied Resistance 167

Glossary 173

Notes 177

Bibliography 189

Index 197

Acknowledgments 211

About the Author 213

Foreword

Thenmozhi Soundararajan

Breathe.

Will you settle in with me as we prepare to dive into Anjali's loving journey of yoga resistance?

There is a part of me that feels discomfort. I worry for Anjali's safety. I worry for the fragility of those who would weaponize our right as humans to engage in somatic practice, and who would twist the unknown diverse histories of yoga in service of global right-wing movements.

It makes my breath shallow, and it catches in my chest. But I remember to ground.

For breath is the foundation of consent. It is the connection between conscious and unconscious thought. And as long as we have breath, we can choose our response and the action that comes forward.

But I still have breath, and so do you. So maybe we can breathe again. And be here. Right now.

And remember, the path for integration is also the path for freedom. Anjali's book is a beautiful and necessary reconciliation of yoga's history and a fertile ground for all of us to reimagine what our practice can grow into today.

This book will provoke you.

It might challenge what you've learned from yoga lineages, your family, or even your country.

But it is important to free yoga from the shackles of ideological history and the dogmatism of Brahminism.

We stretch to release our fascia, settle our nervous systems, and heighten our consciousness.

So too must we stretch and reach for reconciliation of historical harms and generations of caste, religious, and gender violence. As Anjali says, "If we study those who have defied caste and religious norms throughout the history of yoga, we can derive inspiration, healing, and confidence in the changes we must enact as we work to build an inclusive vision of yoga that centers caste abolition, gender equity, and racial justice. . .Knowing about ourselves as human beings who are capable of great love, but who can also inflict great harm on each other, is even more important—and the dire need of our times—when there is war and violence in the name of religion."

This book is doing many things, but two of the most important are: deauthorizing the harmful ideology of Brahminism, which has attempted to appropriate centuries of interfaith and diverse yoga practices; and helping us open a dialogue with members of communities harmed by Brahminism, to cocreate new, shared visions of a liberatory yoga practice rooted in a new understanding of yoga's complex history.

This is not easy.

Dogmatism and orthodoxy are a cancer in yoga training. But I want to ask us: How can there be one way when there are infinite types of bodies, minds, and spirits?

If yoga has many meanings across its schools and lineages, then perhaps the definition I would like to offer is that yoga is a form of knowing —knowing how your body, mind, and spirit integrate.

Say this with me, and then breathe:

Yoga does not belong to one religion, one body type, one language, or one people. Rather, integrative practice is our birthright, and we must lean into inclusion and repair.

I believe you may read this book many times—once to absorb the knowledge intellectually, and again to consider how to incorporate its lessons into your own yoga practice.

This book offers a departure from the typical structure of most yoga teacher trainings, which often reinforce a dominant-caste cis-het male lineage holder who asserts authority without fostering spaces for inquiry, discussion, or dissent. Instead, it presents a gentle, engaging conversation, inviting you as the reader to be an active participant in the exploration Anjali lays out. It revisits traditional ideas while opening pathways for complex, contradictory discourse—not to make proclamations, but to encourage critical inquiry. Ultimately, it is a loving conversation that leaves us better for having engaged with it.

This is how good books work.

This is also how good yoga practice works: revisiting old positions and continually exploring what must be released, reconsidered, and opened. Use that same philosophy with what you learn here.

Read with an open mind and heart. It's okay to disagree, but commit to the discourse. There were moments in the text that created significant dissonance for me. Consider the challenge of engaging with some of the texts discussed in the book. These works are beloved by some, including Anjali, yet they are also responsible for the dehumanization of millions across history. How do we reconcile this? How can we, in our differing experiences, find the regulation and understanding needed to share space, share breath, and ultimately share the world with one another?

This may be the greatest challenge of our generation. It's not unique to yoga communities, but we have the potential to model how to navigate this for others. In moments of dissonance, I found that using my breath to slow down, listen, and seek a shared perspective helped me engage more fully. I hope you will do the same. We can disagree and still learn from one another, remaining in dialogue and connection.

Has yoga always embodied resistance? No. In fact, it has often been stolen from oppressed communities, used to exclude many, and weaponized to support nationalist agendas. But does it have to be this? Absolutely not.

It is our work now to build the practice and the sanghas we need. If extremists try to weaponize yoga, let us liberate it. And liberate ourselves. Let us bring everyone home. And let us heal together.

With deep bows.

Thank you, and let us begin.

Introduction

The past is not static, that which happened long ago; rather, the past carries into the present and shapes our inner and outer lives. It lives on in the air we breathe, the light we carry, and the shadows we bury within. It forms the foundation of policies, the framework of institutions, and the moral fabric of society. From curricula to policy making, national constitutions to popular culture, yoga to religious identity, our narratives of who we are now are based on what we think we know of the past. We learn our values and beliefs from what we have been taught by our parents, teachers, peers, and community. The constructs of what we consider good and bad, right and wrong, failure and success, beautiful and ugly are animated by what is valued, preserved, and mythologized by history. These values in turn form and inform institutions. Thus, history is a dynamic process of rememberings that surface again and again in our conscious and subconscious self.

The past is present.[1] There is a reconstruction or manipulation of past events and texts to lend credence to contemporary dynamics of power and to legitimize ownership of land and culture. The meaning of a word like *dharma*, for instance, has been used, misused, and abused in myriad ways throughout history. A text such as the Bhagavad Gita is used to motivate ancient warriors, inspire anticolonial revolutionaries, uphold the caste system, offer solace to Robert Oppenheimer (the maker of the atomic bomb),[2] and move the everyday practitioner to bhakti. Thus, language, texts, religions, and yoga emerge from specific sociopolitical contexts, meander and shift shapes to suit worldly desires as well as to inform the pursuit of spiritual liberation.

Yoga history is a composite of numerous histories, rooted in a civilization preceding recorded history. There are many approaches to studying yoga history, which spans (arguably and approximately) 2,500 years. During this time there have been tremendous changes in cultures, economies, and politics. Yoga has veritably been a part of the formation of nation-states and the dissolution of civilizations. One could present facts, figures, and periods, or one could delve into texts, art, or archaeology for information on yoga. While scholars have paved inroads into a dense corpus of yoga history, the scholarship has been largely academic and hence daunting for the everyday practitioner.

History is not a presentation of neutral and objective information. It is more than people, dates, and places; it is who gets to record the events and how that information is explained by the historians (historiography). Historical data is influenced by the historian's sociocultural-political background. History often has an embedded bias. The ones who record and inscribe are the ones who have the power and resources to do so. Since it was mostly cis men who had access to writing and recording events, there was a "serious distortion of the record of civilization" and a perception that "men devised theories and explanatory systems of thought; women took care of the rearing of children, domestic production, and the maintenance of daily life. These false assertions led to the equally erroneous claim that women had no history, or at least no history worth recording."[3]

This book crystallizes invisible interstices of power, often unnamed or unspoken in yoga spaces. There is a need not only to understand the historical and sociological contexts of the texts and teachings, but also to study how yoga has been and is being co-opted by orthodoxy and nationalism. Insight into these complexities can be integral to building solidarity with folks who are actively encountering these harmful systems. If we study those who have defied caste and religious norms throughout the history of yoga, we can derive inspiration, healing, and confidence in the changes we must enact as we work to build an inclusive vision of yoga that centers caste abolition, gender equity, and racial justice. If we study those who challenged the construct of gender two thousand years ago, we may feel less alone today in fighting regulations birthed in misogyny, transphobia, and homophobia. The endeavor is to sift through yoga history with the objective of contextualizing some of the integral developments in yoga and to reclaim the echoes of resistance from those in the past who confronted formidable personal and systemic obstacles with ingenuity, grace, and resilience.

I have a quilt with hand-sewn, raggedy stitches in which deep reds wriggle next to mossy greens. This *godhadi*, made from patches of old sarees and leftover fabric, is a warm riot of colors and scraps of different hues and textures. Some of these pieces are rough to the touch, made of hardy cottons, while others are bright, satiny silks. On its own, each scrap does not make much of a statement; nor does it have much functionality. What can one do with a small, square piece of cloth? However, when the scraps are sewn together we get a vibrant, homey comforter and a keepsake of moments represented by beloved sarees. The quilt is an apt metaphor for yoga. Just like the quilt has different colors and textures, some bright and smooth, others dull and rough, yoga has dimensions that illuminate one's potential for liberation and also oppress many. As yoga practitioners, we need to know the many roots of yoga as well as the shadows that conceal the unsavoriness of the past.

Yoga is regarded as a spiritual practice and is not often looked at with a critical lens on the dynamics of power and privilege within the system. From the rather mysterious Patanjali, the composer of the Yoga Sutras, to the more ubiquitous figure of Krishna on a battlefield, we learn about the paths and the practices to expand our awareness of who we are: sovereign and interconnected embodiments of consciousness. Yoga has traversed many winding by-lanes through centuries to be where it is today. Yoga is and always has been embedded within the social context of the times. For some, yoga is a practice of liberation from suffering, of solace and rest, of enlightenment and self-realization. For others, such as those impacted by the caste system or religious fundamentalism, much of yoga is oppressive and harmful because they have been willfully excluded and violently kept away from accessing many of the teachings. The long arms of yoga history also have embraced movements of resistance against oppression. A remembrance of these rebellious, resilient voices can inform and inspire our own endeavors of resistance against contemporary dominant cultures. Learning about our history is critical if we want to learn about ourselves. Knowing about ourselves as human beings who are capable of great love, but who can also inflict great harm on each other, is even more important—and the dire need of our times—when there is war and violence in the name of religion.

Reexamining Yoga's History

A reclamation of yoga histories is important, especially as yoga is subsumed by the interplay of a few -isms, primarily neoliberal spiritual capitalism, which I define here as a system that emphasizes individual responsibility for one's own health, happiness, and well-being while ignoring systemic inequities of class, gender, race, caste, and ability. This individualistic orientation of self-care ensures the preservation of the status quo through "applications of spirituality that concentrate on healing the broken person rather than undermining the system that broke that person in the first place."[4] According to this paradigm, the onus is on the individual to self-regulate and self-govern to optimize performance, participation, and consumption in a capitalistic economy. Neoliberal spiritual industries sell goods and practices that offer quick Band-Aid solutions to systemic and institutional problems. They do not empower individuals in any democratic sense but impose new modes of governance. According to Andrea Jain, professor of religious studies, they maintain "social hierarchies in which those who attain perfection through these modes are and remain at the top."[5]

Neoliberal spiritual capitalism facilitates a concerted consumption of goods and practices framed as conscious and righteous self-care. It soothes a harrowed twenty-first-century society on the precipice of climate crises, ongoing wars and genocides, and the glaring disparities of wealth without challenging the inequities created by race, class, gender, ability, and caste. Yoga has been a prominent component in popular self-care culture since the latter part of the twentieth century due to a variety of reasons, including the great successes of yoga gurus, exoticization of "Eastern spirituality," and emphasis on Euro-patriarchal beauty ideals of thinness. Yoga's popularity grew with burgeoning middle- and urban-class elites and is now mostly known as a health and fitness modality. It has become big business: "American yoga practitioners alone reported spending over $16 billion on yoga apparel, equipment, classes, and other accoutrements in 2016."[6] Most practitioners of yoga do not know of its long history, or that it even has a history. The distinct traditions of yoga have been hybridized and reduced to a mostly physical practice on the mat, undermining its multidimensional, pluralistic, and sometimes countercultural histories. Reductiveness ensures a pseudouniformity, making capitalistic manipulations easier—it is easier to sell simple things and practices rather than to delve into cultural complexities.

Neoliberal spirituality is prevalent across the globe. Baba Ramdev, India's most well-known yoga guru, is the cofounder and CEO of a company named Patanjali Ayurved that has over two hundred thousand outlets and grossed over $1.5 billion in 2017.[7] Patanjali Ayurved sells a wide range of products—such as toothpaste, *atta* (wheat flour) noodles, breakfast cereals, and many other items—that they advertise as "natural food products," "natural health care," and "natural personal care." Their vision statement says they aim to keep "Nationalism, Ayurved and Yog[a] as our pillars," thus blending a heady smorgasbord of patriotism, health, and consumerism.[8] Ramdev has also touted yoga as a "cure for homosexuality"[9] and campaigned for criminalizing homosexuality in 2009 after the Delhi High Court ruled in favor of decriminalization. He is a close advisor of India's prime minister, Narendra Modi, and this brings us to the other -ism in yoga: religious nationalism, or Hindutva, translated as the essence of Hindu or Hinduness.

Hindutva and Yoga

Hindutva is premised on otherization[10] in which all entities, particularly Muslims, are framed as antagonistic to the Hindus, whom Hindutva adherents believe are the original inhabitants of India. This communal worldview privileges a dominant caste and hypermasculine ideology. It was first developed by Savarkar as a nationalist anticolonial resistance and developed by the Rashtriya Swayamsevak Sangh, a paramilitary anticolonial voluntary organization founded by K. B. Hedgewar in 1925 on the premise that "Hindu culture is the life-breath of Hindusthan,"[11] another name for India. The Hindutva ideology imposes a homogeneity upon a historically profusely diverse land of cultures, languages, religions, and belief systems, and it centers the idea of a modern India as a Hindu *rashtra* (nation). It is an inherently exclusionary process that endorsed violent resistance against British colonialism, and in the context of contemporary India it "indicates the extent to which patriarchy, gendered ideologies . . . as well as the sacredness of Sanskrit define the predominant understanding of the identity of a Hindu."[12]

Prime Minister Narendra Modi is the current face of the Hindutva movement. He is also a self-professed yoga enthusiast whose first official act after taking office in 2014 was to propose to the United Nations that the world should observe an International Day of Yoga. In his petition to the UN, he said: "Yoga embodies unity of mind and body; thought and action; restraint and fulfillment; harmony between man and nature; a holistic approach to health and well-being. It is not about exercise, but discover[ing] the sense of oneness with yourself, the world and nature."[13]

Modi's petition was signed by 175 countries,[14] and the first International Day of Yoga was held in 2015. In New Delhi Modi led a televised practice for thirty-nine thousand people from eighty-four countries, which set two Guinness world records. Modi's image of a peace-loving yoga practitioner is in sharp contrast to the anti-Muslim rhetoric of his campaign speeches, where he often calls Muslims "infiltrators,"[15] as well as the decline of the rights of women and gender, caste, and religious minorities in India.[16] India's ranking in the Human Freedom Index is 110 out of 165 countries.[17] Under the government's strict sedition and counterterrorism laws, such as the Public Safety Act and the Unlawful Activities Prevention Act,[18] dissenters, protesting farmers, marginalized groups such as the Dalits, and minority religions such as Sikhs, Muslims, and others have been threatened, arrested, and harmed when speaking out against the government's actions. The co-optation of yoga as a soft power is a political tool to strategically homogenize a diverse culture and is part of the "om-washing" of "a radical agenda of ethno-nationalist state violence," according to sociologist and yoga teacher Dr. Sheena Sood.[19]

"Hindu nationalists reduce yoga's complex formative history to promote the ideals of Brahminical Hinduism, appropriating and erasing yoga's connections to Buddhist, Sufi, Jain, and Tantric traditions in South Asia," says Angana Chatterji, a human rights activist and scholar at the University of California, Berkeley, who has written extensively on Hindu nationalism.[20] The Hindutva's notion of yoga is cisheteronormative and amplifies casteist hierarchies without an acknowledgement of the diverse and pluralistic streams in yoga history.

Religious nationalism is rooted in communal and colonial understandings of history that necessitate categorization of peoples with rigid boundaries, creating an "us" versus "them." It is important to note that all major religions and traditions—Islam, Christianity, Judaism—have extremist elements and essentialist tendencies. The scope of this book and my expertise is limited to unraveling a few of the threads as it pertains to yoga. In the context of yoga, the communal interpretation of history underlines Sanskrit as the root language of Indic thought and that yoga is a Hindu practice. These are interrelated claims and stem from a particular orthodox narrative that does not consider (or has subsumed) heterodoxical traditions and praxis. In reality, and as we'll see in the coming chapters, Hinduism is a composite of many sociocultural-political elements. Yoga overlaps and interacts with this composite in many ways. The intersections are not very clear to the modern yoga practitioner, who is taught that yoga comes from India, and India is conflated with Hindu, thus yoga is Hindu.

Yoga is not a singular practice; rather, it is an amalgamation of many often-divergent philosophies, traditions, and cultures. The development of yoga stems from an intermingling of different threads. Some of these strands, like caste, are invisible, and others are more visible. Yoga has adapted and mutated in complex ways from its ascetic roots to the householder traditions to incorporation of devotional movements to the transnational body-centric phenomenon it is today.

Hindutva claims that yoga is a Hindu practice. The Take Back Yoga campaign, organized by the Hindu American Foundation, emphasized that "yoga is a spiritual discipline rooted in Hindu philosophy and is universally available to anyone without any coercion, pressure, or requirement to change one's religion."[21] The organization further shares references about yoga from the Upanishads, the Bhagavad Gita, and the Yoga Sutras, along with quotes from teachers like Swami Vivekananda, B. K. S. Iyengar, and Pattabhi Jois. The campaign was a response to a 2013 lawsuit filed by parents in Encinitas, California, to stop yoga in the schools because they believed that yoga had religious overtones and it was promoting Hinduism.[22] While it is important to call out the lawsuit's undercurrents of xenophobia, it is also imperative to explicate the central discourse of the response. There is a conflation of yoga with one stream of "Hindu" philosophy. The multidimensional tapestry of yoga includes many other threads from different religious, philosophical, and cultural sources.

History teaches us that truths are many, contradictions and paradoxes abound, and past relationships between religions, castes, ethnicities, genders, and nations were far more dynamic and fluid than what we know today. Knowing about these pluralistic and synergistic roots is especially important when there is an imposition of reductive versions of both yoga and Hinduism. While many in the West are perhaps more aware about cultural appropriation, we are less cognizant of the heterodoxical traditions and resistance movements that are a part of the evolution of yoga. The umbrella of yoga also includes the historical appropriation and absorption of varied cultural beliefs, traditions, ideologies, and religions. Thus, we need to move beyond the binaries of appropriation versus appreciation and situate the discussion within the dynamics of power, historical context, cultural understandings, and socioeconomic realities.

Ethnonationalist ideologies homogenize even where heterogeneity thrives, a stark contradiction to the deep heterodoxy of diverse thought traditions and philosophical systems that in turn shaped the container of yoga. In the first millennium BCE, Buddhists, Jains, agnostics, and atheists competed with adherents of what we now call Hinduism.[23] The renunciate *sramana*s rejected the ritualistic rigidity and hierarchy of Vedic religion, and in its stead they emphasized self-realization and ahimsa, the principle of the nonharming of all beings, human and nonhuman. The Charvakas were materialists who challenged both the sramanic belief in rebirth and the Vedic appeasement of gods. The Bhakti movement consisted of spontaneous and radical uprisings that disrupted caste, patriarchy, and rigidity of religious affiliations. Heterodoxy was generative and produced a rich and dynamic repertoire of values, traditions, and cultures that have shaped yoga.

Yoga is situated in the larger Indic culture and is not a monolith. Cultures are never homogenous, unalloyed, or static; there is no pristine, pure culture that continues as such throughout history.[24] Since we will be exploring the impact of orthodoxy, it is important to define the term more explicitly. Orthodoxy in this context is an acceptance and regard of the centrality of Vedic literature and Brahmanic religion as a "standard against which all other traditions and orientations are measured."[25] Vedic literature was composed in Sanskrit, a language accessible mostly to Brahmin men, encapsulating what they deemed important. Thus, the Vedic canon elucidates philosophies and histories from a particular worldview, but it certainly does not include all other positionalities. Colonial scholars and lawmakers amplified some of these texts and further institutionalized caste-based stratifications. Over the centuries, Brahmanical orthodoxy—sometimes also referred to as Vedic Brahmanism—emerged as the dominant religion and impacted spiritual and religious phenomena, including yoga. We will explore some of the main constituents of Vedic literature and Brahmanic religion in the next chapter.

The roots of yoga were birthed in orthodoxy as well as its opposite paradigm, heterodoxy. Heterodoxy is deviation from orthodoxy, and yet these radical aspects of yoga got absorbed by dominant Brahmanical traditions. Deviation from normative orthodoxy also generated new religious and spiritual traditions. These movements—some huge, moving and impacting millions, and some tiny, creating ripples of change in their communities— were mostly led or created by marginalized people who discarded repressive threads such as caste, patriarchy, and dogma. Some crossed boundaries of gender, geography, and religion, while others attempted to innovate and fuse ideas and praxis. Contrary to the trope of yoga as a peaceful "Zen" practice unperturbed by the trials and tribulations of the world, the traditions of yoga included vociferous debate, radical dissent, loving devotion, and violent and nonviolent resistance as direct and bold confrontations of orthodoxy. Each of the four stories shared in the upcoming chapters will highlight these different pathways—voices of the ancients that we need to heed today in our courageous work of challenging oppression.

The chapters ahead will first define some key terms like *yoga* and *Hindu* and will contextualize orthodoxy. Each of these claims will be unpacked with insight into heterodoxy as resistance by uplifting radical feminist narratives. We will chisel away at hierarchical categories as we delve into questions regarding the constructs of caste and gender in yoga and the coexistence of sexuality, sensuality, and spirituality. These issues are often refracted through a Brahmanical lens, left unsaid or considered unimportant in orthodox narratives. We blur these rigid boundaries not to confound and confuse, but to clarify that all of us are not one or the other; we are instead both wildly, imperfectly human and deeply sacred beings.

Yoga is the science and the art of seeking liberation. While radical asceticism was a part of the practices of ancient seekers (known as rishis), there are other pathways. These traditions are often embodied by practitioners who challenge dominant narratives, and yoga scholars haven't delved into them with as much rigor and gusto for many reasons—mostly the dominance of patriarchy. Many of the nonconformist, subversive elements of varied yoga traditions have been lost, erased, or greatly diminished. It is my humble hope that these narratives of resistance will lead to more curiosity about the past and how the present is shaped by the foibles as well as the epiphanies of our ancestors.

A Note on Method, Scope, Positionality, and Language

As a yoga practitioner who grew up in India in a Hindu family, I studied the Bhagavad Gita in a community center under the tutelage of a young priest who impressed his teenage students with his charm and devotion. My mother often told us that a prayer was a conversation with God. It does not have to be an elaborate display; rather, it is a heartfelt connection. I believed her. Faith was a soothing salve during turbulent times, and an anchor for community, celebration, and joy during others. The deepest visceral connection to the divine was through dance expressed through *abhinaya* (facial expression) and mudras (gestures) accompanied by songs composed by seekers of truth and liberation. I found solace in chanting the one thousand names of Devi and Vishnu when I was undergoing surgery for early-stage breast cancer. I loved (and still love) going to old temples and marveling at the intricate architecture. Bhakti was my way of naming and remembering the sacred, seeking connections, inside and out. I was not particularly ritualistic. Like so many of us who grew up in the 1980 and 1990s in larger Indian metropolitan cities, I was educated in Catholic institutions that were informed and influenced by the British. There was always a struggle to determine what it means to be a Hindu and an Indian in postcolonial India. However, there was not much understanding of caste privilege.

While I rebelled against prevalent societal taboos against intercaste marriages, rejected the implicit and explicit patriarchy of the *upanayam* (a Brahmin ritual of initiation with a thread that was for boys only), and questioned the depictions and predicaments of folks like Shumbaka, Shurpanaka, and Ekalavya in epic literature, my deconstruction of what it means to be a Hindu has been gradual—and yes, even painful. As my own study and practice of yoga deepened, I began to see the interweaving threads of Brahminism and patriarchy that course through some of the teachings. I became more aware of the range of variants of a text like the Ramayana or the different portrayals of Radha. I studied the works of Dr. Bhimrao Ambedkar, Jyotirao Phule, and Gail Omvedt, and of historians such as Uma Chakravarti and Romila Thapar, and I followed the work of caste abolitionists based in the United States like Thenmozhi Soundararajan and Prachi Patankar. It dawned on me that Hindu teachings were not universally liberatory, that there were dimensions that were oppressive, and that caste discrimination and violence is very much alive in the diaspora.

I began to inquire into the histories of texts. Who were the people who composed and narrated these different retellings? What were their positionalities of caste and gender? What were their motivations and aspirations? What messages about social obligations and gender norms are embedded within the texts? How was the "other" constructed in the great epics? How do these constructions inform and form past and present sociopolitical discourse? In yoga spaces I have often witnessed many shades of silence, diffidence, and defiance among yoga practitioners and educators when there is a mention of caste and religion, or when someone discusses how some of the teachings of yoga texts, such as *Hatha Yoga Pradipika*, are blatantly misogynistic by modern standards. The responses run the gamut of either quoting other caste-privileged pandits or asserting that mentions of *varna-jaatis* (i.e., class and caste) in the Bhagavad Gita are symbolic representations of esoteric concepts. There is a denial that such teachings have resonance and impact in the material and socioemotional lives of many who are caste oppressed.

Yoga today is perceived mostly as a fitness and wellness modality, targeted toward the elite, white, and able-bodied cis woman. From goat yoga to paddleboard yoga to hot yoga and power yoga, there is a reductionism of the liberatory potential of yoga in the modern world. I witness this in India too, in the burgeoning numbers of gymnasiums that offer yoga as a fitness modality; the reductive version of yoga has been exported back to the roots of its origins. From bookshelves to conferences, from teaching jobs to access to yoga classes, there is an exclusion of marginalized communities, including the erasure of South Asian teachers. This is one of the many reasons that there is a diffidence and silence about caste oppression among South Asian practitioners.

Another reason needs a more thorough unpacking and stems from a long history of institutional sanctioning of caste, patriarchy, and their intersections. Yoga texts and practices either deny, gloss over, or are ignorant of the implications of caste narratives. Therefore, discernment is critical, with an acknowledgement that the teachings are embedded in the context of the times, reflecting values, norms, and hierarchies, with a plethora of interpretations and retellings. There are also multiple dimensions of meaning in a myth, epic, or text. Some of the different approaches are the four levels of analysis of myth put forward by Lévi-Strauss: "the narrative level of the story, the metaphorical level as a struggle between gods and demons, the cosmic level of metaphysical principles and symbolic truths, and the human level of the search for meaning in human life."[26]

For example, in the Mahabharata, one may understand Arjuna as a representation for all human beings, dejected and confused about how right action is actualized (the human level). Or we may understand Arjuna as the embodiment of the *guna* of *rajas*, the attribute of action, according to Samkhya philosophy (the cosmic level); or we may even understand Arjuna as the individual consciousness (*jivatma*). There is also a sociological level, Arjuna as a Kshatriya, the warrior-prince whose dharma (duty/obligation) is to fight the war even if it means killing his own kith and kin. In the Mahabharata, dharma is explained as the ways and means of upholding the duties of one's *varna* and annihilating all that gets in the way, like the demand for the Nishada tribal prince, Ekalavya, to sacrifice his thumb. Even if that story was added in later versions of the epic, as is often asserted by *savarna*s (those who are within the *varna* system, and thus privileged), it means that at the time of the addition and retelling, there was a social hierarchy being formulated and established.

If you are a caste-privileged practitioner, as I am, you can interrogate how you understand and internalize the norms and the values embedded in teachings. If you are a non–South Asian practitioner, I invite you to reflect on the ways you hold structural and systemic privilege. Tracing our own deeply ingrained *samskaras* (patterns of thought and behavior) is unsettling to say the least, as it reveals ancestral and present traumas. I am aware of being both an oppressor, as a savarna, and the oppressed, as a colonized and racialized being. It is an iterative process that entails an unraveling that cannot be rushed and yet forms the very essence of resistance. As you read, I invite you to notice when there is discomfort or dissonance and turn to the practices of embodiment that yoga offers. As practitioners, we know how discomfort feels in our bodies, in our breath, where we hold tension and how we can invite more ease as we seek *vidya*, perennial truths, beyond the constraints of our cultural conditionings, *avidya*.

This is the work of individual and collective transformation, the inner work that can ignite the outer work, pivotal to dismantle oppression, both within and without. Many questions and doubts may surface about our own long-held beliefs and value systems, even our identities. I am even now tussling with a few of my own: How is my faith, my bhakti, truly liberatory and loving? How do I chant in Sanskrit, a practice that gives me much solace, when I know the complex history of Sanskrit? I often turn to the teachings of nonattachment, *vairagya*. I share this to be transparent about not only my positionality but also my own lifelong and ongoing processes of unlearning and relearning, and to offer some of my personal reflections in the hope that it aids you in finding your own path. I share all this with a humility that stems from the excavations of my positionality as a cis savarna who questioned these systems as a child growing up in Bangalore, India.

I use translations of three texts as primary sources: Bhagavad Gita, Manu Smriti, and *Gita Govinda*. The other texts I consult are secondary sources from specialists in source texts like the Vedas, the Mahabharata, the Ramayana, and the Upanishads, and from trained historians who dive into philosophy, philology, historical linguistics, archaeology, sociology, religious studies, and ethnography. In particular I am grateful for the scholarship of Romila Thapar, Ruth Vanita, Arti Dhand, Uma Chakravarti, and Anshu

Malhotra. Although I have studied Sanskrit, I am not a Sanskritist, so I have shared translations from acclaimed Sanskrit scholars when needed.

I use binary pronouns for mythical and historical figures based on how they have been referred to in texts, which may not be their entire truth. This is a limitation of language, cisheteronormativity, and historical studies, and it needs to be named as such because it contributes to societal bias. Women and men include trans and cis folks. In addition, Tristan Katz, facilitator in topics related to LGBTQ+ topics and diversity, equity, and inclusion, reminds us that we also need to acknowledge that "grouping non-binary people with binary identities is harmful."[27] Gender expansiveness is a part of yogic teaching that will be explored in chapter 3.

My approach is that of a storyteller in the rich *kathaka* storytelling traditions of South Asia. In each chapter, I use a character or a person from one of the following specific time periods—Upanishadic, Puranic, Bhakti, and colonial—to spark curiosity about further explorations of the multidimensional and heterodox aspects of yoga history. These are periods when there were seismic shifts in collective social consciousness that led to reformulations of religion and caste that in turn shaped the expansive repository of yoga. The scope of the work is limited to the topics mentioned in the earlier section of this chapter. The stories and the issues span centuries; thus it is a primer for deeper study and reflection. The book does not detail all feminist historical narratives or stories, but it does address some important ones. This is not a comprehensive history of yoga, India, or Hinduism, and it doesn't detail every historical landmark or delve into every aspect of patriarchy. Rather, it is a panoramic view of yoga that weaves narratives often overlooked in yoga studies, and it discusses how these stories can inspire and inform the present moment.

Radical Storytelling as a Disruptive Practice

I come from a land of a billion stories. I dream often of the warm lap of my grandmother, her sturdy arms holding me gently, and her rather raspy voice bearing tales of bygone times when the gods and goddesses walked among us mortals. She was a good storyteller, vivid in her descriptions of the land, the verdant forests, the village deities who were fierce guardians of all beings, human and nonhuman. She spoke in our native language, Konkani, about beings who lived in this world and other worlds. These narrations are also lessons in how we can be dedicated in pursuit of liberation, overcome all sorts of obstacles, and be in right relationship with each other. These stories are a composite of imagination and reality, myth and history, aspiration and pragmatism, teaching us everything under the sun and beyond about love and loss, victory and defeat, good and evil, matter and spirit, mind and body, death and immortality. Thus, I turn to her, to my ancestors, to a whole lineage of storytellers.

In Sanskrit, the word *itihasa*—which translates to "it was indeed like that"—refers to subjective narrative accounts of events, rather than a chronological, factual account of dates and people. This approach underlines that the past is known vis-à-vis specific lenses, so these stories are not absolute truths. The history of yoga does not lend itself to a linear, chronological narrative, because "it" evolved in a scattered, diffused way all over the ancient Indic region. One can describe yoga by using the metaphor of an ocean. The ocean is vast and touches upon different shores. Each of these shores has a landscape and a unique ecosystem. Yoga is like that ocean that touches the shores of time. Each period has contributions from the development of sociopolitical systems such as nation-states, caste, religion, and capitalism. We need to delve into this long, checkered history to understand the less savory aspects of yoga and learn about the systems of patriarchy, caste, and imperialism that shaped its development—systems that continue to be leveraged by nationalist forces today. These systemic hierarchies operate in every realm, from material access to resources to the more spiritual longings of all human beings for transcendence. Many of these histories are unknown in mainstream yoga. Those who do know some of them do not know how to receive and metabolize the underbelly of yoga's past and how it manifests in the present.

The teachings of yoga were conveyed through storytelling. These stories, in addition to being informative and laden with insight into the human experience, are chronicles of the times that shed light on the sociopolitical interplay of gender, caste, and religion. For example, a collection of stories called *Mahabuddhavamsa*—composed in Pali (a language more accessible than Sanskrit) around the second century BCE—was a hagiography of the many births of Buddha. The Jataka tales assimilated regional fables to share Buddhist teachings. The Upanishads used stories to discuss the nature of abstract perennial reality, or the Brahman. The Puranas are a treasure trove of tales of the divine given physical form and personhood, such as Ganesha, Vishnu, and Devi. Vedic tenets like dharma and moksha were reinforced through conversations and situations in the Mahabharata and the Ramayana. The Bhagavad Gita, considered as one of the most influential spiritual teachings in the world, is embedded in the Mahabharata, one of two epics of ancient India.

Mythological, historical, and fictional accounts of human relationships are ways in which we practice empathy, compassion, and conflict. Ancients have narrated stories under trees and starry skies, on battlefields, and in *gurukuls* (forest universities). These tales explain great spiritual truths and bear wise messages about the complexity and nuances of the human experience. Narratives shine a light onto the dynamics of power and who and what is considered to be valuable. Stories breathe life into the past and connect our vast humanity across generations. Storytelling was one of the integral methods for sharing esoteric and abstract concepts in ways that were relatable to ordinary people living ordinary lives. Rich, complex narratives were woven around fundamental questions such as the nature of reality, the concept of consciousness, the purpose of human life, and the complexities of being engaged in the world as social beings. The characters in the stories from the Puranas and epic literature traversed liminal spaces between humanity and divinity.

The orality of the storytelling traditions ensures a porousness as narrations move through regions and generations, absorbing the sociopolitical and cultural ethos of the times. We also find similarities among stories from Hinduism, Buddhism, and Jainism because all these three religions underwent development and shifts around the same time. Ideas, concepts, and archetypes flowed from one religion to the other. Indra, the chief Vedic god associated with thunder and lightning, also appears in Buddhist mythology as a lesser powerful deity. While storytelling was and continues to be a crucial component of Indic culture, there is a fluid tension between village/regional narrative traditions and the pan-Hindu traditions. There is a reflexivity[28] that generates new traditions out of old ones, producing families of texts in different languages and dialects as deities were absorbed from regional clans/tribes (*kulas*) into wider "classical" or Sanskritic forms. This also was not a one-way process. For instance, Draupadi, the polyandrous wife of the Pandavas of the Mahabharata, gets worshipped as a Parashakti who is also the Great Goddess[29] in a Tamil folk tradition that can be traced to the thirteenth century in the Gingee region (modern Arcot in Tamil Nadu). Even today she is worshipped in temples and in ritual enactments in *terukkūttu*s (street dramas) that culminate in *timiti*, a spectacular fire walk in which Draupadi Devi accompanies devotees, fulfilling their wishes.

The text, therefore, is not "a repository of timeless truth" but rather "a temporally conditioned object."[30] It is not a static product; rather, it is a dynamic process that can change and evolve into different forms. The teachings of yoga are embedded in multiple versions of these texts, not just one. This is an important consideration, especially now when there is a concerted effort to present an ossified pan-Hindu, dominant-caste perspective for political maneuverings. Hence it is important for us as discerning yoga practitioners to know the evolutions and the sources of ideas, stories, and symbols so we can expand our own understandings of the human and the divine.

Embodied Resistance, Sacred Resilience

Resistance is embodied. Embodiment is a fundamental human need, and yet in the modern world we often feel disembodied. We live and learn increasingly through virtual media, through screens rather than in contact, in touch with the earth, with our neighbors, with ourselves. This gives rise to a disconnection with our inner truths, and it leads to dehumanizing the "other." Disembodiment leads to dysregulated reactions rather than intentional responses to the world within us and around us. The stories in this book foreground embodied resistance in different periods in yoga history in the hope that they inspire and inform you as we face an unprecedented rise in patriarchy, racism, and nationalism all over the world.

Resilience is sacred. By sacred I mean integral and principled, rather than canonized or idealized. Each of the stories in this book portrays forms of resistance, resilience, and dissent in unique ways. Some mock and tear down constructs of power with a fierce intellectual vociferousness, while others do so with bhakti, the radical and revolutionary love of the divine. They reveal the kaleidoscopic nature of humanity while seeking salvation. They challenge the notion that a spiritual aspirant must be cauterized from seeking pleasure and sensuality.

Each chapter delves into topics that are either ignored, glossed over, denied, or erased in mainstream yoga spaces that reinforce and replay a homogeneity of dominant cultures and ethnonationalist political agendas. The stories lead us into explorations of issues like gender expansiveness, the continuum of sexuality and spirituality, and the fluidity between castes and religions. Some of them are known, and others need to be more known by everyday practitioners, not just scholars and researchers. I believe the more we hear of these wayward, radical, rebellious beings, the better it is for the seekers of liberation today. Some of them were revered during their lifetime, while others were reviled for their daring blasphemy. Some of them renounced their attachment to the body, others flourished in eros, and yet others transcended body and gender with a shameless, full-blooded, searing embrace of the sacred.

The first two chapters detail some of the fundamental questions such as the numerous definitions of yoga and the identities of the people who composed the Vedas. Questions regarding the origin of yoga, the concept of Indigeneity, the foundation of the caste system are important for us to unravel because they are highly controversial, and they form the bases of politically charged conflicts and claims that India and yoga are "originally Hindu." The book focuses on these root inquiries rather than relating an all-encompassing history of the Hindus or the Indian subcontinent.

The next four chapters start with a story from a specific period or that has been birthed through the collective imaginations of the peoples from that period. Chapter 3 begins with a story of Sulabha, the scholar-ascetic from the Vedic period, and her debate with King Janaka. Using this story as a springboard, there is a discussion on the construct and dynamics of gender, and a framework for locating gender histories that will be used in the ensuing chapters.

Chapter 4 reimagines the story of Radha and Krishna as an inquiry into the inherent paradoxes between spirituality and sensuality, building on the framework of the previous chapter. Radha's story demystifies her metamorphosis from a tribal heroine to being worshipped as a goddess-consort of the Hindu pantheon.

Chapter 5 leads with a story about Akka Mahadevi, the prolific twelfth-century Bhakti poet who defied gender and caste norms with her unabashed devotion to Shiva. We examine the dynamic tension between major religions of the time, and we explore the complexities of bhakti and the Bhakti movement.

Chapter 6 introduces Piro, a nineteenth-century Muslim courtesan from Punjab, who fiercely reclaimed autonomy regarding her narrative and wrote an autobiographical account as a Gulabdasi, which was a heterodox sect integrating aspects of Sufi, Sikh, and Vedantic thought. At the end of chapters 3, 4, 5, and 6 are considerations for ongoing reflection, study, and practice, with the intention that it helps all of us—as practitioners and as socially conscious beings—to be courageous in our disruption of patriarchy, casteism, and the rhetoric of separatist ethnonationalism that plagues the world today.

The conclusion delves into the ways in which we can be discerning yoga practitioners in contemporary times in solidarity with caste abolitionists, disrupt the harmful impact of religious hegemony, and truly ensure that we can build spaces of healing and liberation for all.

May these stories ignite a radical reimagination of our communities.

May we be courageous in our questions of what is and vulnerable in our answers of what could be.

May the truths of our ancestors light our paths to cogenerate collective liberation.

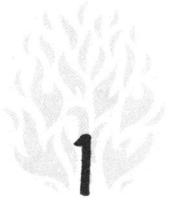

1

ORIGINS OF YOGA
AND HINDUISM

The head of a unicorn thrusts itself out of the emptiness, virile,
arched, and alive. The enclosed space is the womb, the vessel of
energy, from which life becomes manifest. The spaces created by
the arms of the six limbed form are fluid, suggesting the expanding
and contracting of a live organism. The movement of the Eka-
Sringi, the mythical unicorn, is against the sun; the head points
backwards. The seal from Mohenjo-Daro is a mandala of supreme
magic, a paradigm that reveals the circular rhythm of birth and
dissolution and the awesome secrets of transformation.

—PUPUL JAYAKAR, *The Earthen Drum*

Let's begin at the very beginning. One of the issues that is greatly politicized
today is concerned with the identities of the "original inhabitants" of India,
who, it is claimed, were the originators of yoga. The chapter delves into this
complex query. The winding story of ancient India weaves through multiple
waves of migrations, invasions, and intermingling, with great conflicts as well as
prosaic coexistence. Each wave of migrants commingled with previous inhabitants, producing new cultures, varied ways of living, and diverse traditions.

The Hindutva assertion that the original people of the land that is now
known as India were Hindus and that everyone else was the foreign other

is, at best, simplistic. It is centered around Brahmanical orthodoxy, which posits that the Vedic people were Indigenous to the land and practiced a utopian way of life, a *sanatan* (eternal) dharma, until disruption from Islamic invaders and European colonization. According to this ideology, the people who practiced this dharma also birthed and practiced yoga. Moreover, there is an assertion that the Vedic period was the golden age of India, an emphatic proselytization of the eternality of Vedic wisdom.

There is a claim that the Vedas were authorless (*a-paurusheya*), deeming them as sacred literature and hence above mortal critique. During the Vedic time, we are told, women in India "went beyond traditional roles, married at a mature age and had the right to choose their husbands" until invasions from "outsiders."[1] This mythologized eternality of the existence of Hindus and Indigeneity is often operationalized to impose sociopolitical-cultural hegemony and dominance, because it proclaims other religions (especially Islam and Christianity) to be foreign or alien. In this idealized notion of *sanatan* dharma and ancient yoga, there is very little acknowledgement of heterogeneity, movements of resistance and dissent, or oppressive threads of caste and patriarchy that undeniably also course through the tapestry.

The broad brushstrokes that paint a picture of this period do not reveal the existence of a rich heterodoxy that contributed greatly not only to the teachings of yoga but also to overall human thought and imagination. In addition to the ritual-oriented Vedic Brahmanism—consisting of religious traditions that centered the tenets of the Vedic literature and were oriented around formulations of caste roles—there were parallel traditions that thrived alongside but are not acknowledged as important, and that have been erased or appropriated. There were dissenting perspectives to the existential and soteriological questions that have intrigued humans in languages other than Sanskrit. The sramanas (renunciates), for instance, challenged Vedic Brahmanism and used languages like Pali and Prakrit, which were far more accessible to folks across caste and class. The sramanic traditions later coalesced to form new religious and philosophical traditions like Jainism and Buddhism.

There are many questions that we need to look into to gain a better understanding about the origin of yoga. Most practitioners today acknowledge asanas (poses), pranayama (breath regulation for channeling prana, or breath), and dhyana (meditation) as a wholesome yoga practice, along with study of a few texts like Patanjali's Yoga Sutras, the Bhagavad Gita, and some Upanishads. Some may practice mantra (chants) and mudra (gestures) or *kirtan* (devotional singing), all in the name of yoga, and yet few may know that these practices stem from different traditions that have evolved and shaped each other. Hatha Yoga and Patanjali's Yoga Sutras, for instance, come from different time periods in yoga history and have different emphases. The former is a transmutation of the gross and subtle bodies, while the latter emphasizes the psychological aspect of the mind as a tool for liberating us from attachments to the material/phenomenal world (*prakriti*). Yet both are studied today as a seamless entity. Transnational yoga—i.e., globally practiced yoga—is thus an amalgamation, a composite of multiple, often contradictory traditions and lineages that is vastly different from its ascetic origins. While the west has commodified yoga as a multibillion-dollar industry, reducing it to a fitness modality, the nationalist ideology emphasizes yoga's "Hindu" origins. The scope of this chapter is to set the stage for explorations that go into the roots of patriarchy in Brahmanic religion, rather than to examine the long history of yoga comprehensively.

Laying the Foundation

We are kin, you and I. We are all related, not just in a vague, "spiritual" way but in a genetically provable way. Human life began in Africa; more precisely, the earliest remains of a modern human (three hundred thousand years old), *Homo sapiens*, were found in a cave in Jebel Irhoud in Morocco.[2] We all have a common ancestor. We are all interconnected genetically, spiritually, and culturally, something that we often forget when we wage wars over boundaries and nations in our quest for cultural, political, and economic dominance and hegemony. Around sixty-five thousand years ago, migrants from Africa reached Asia and Europe and encountered a population of archaic humans (members of other *Homo* species). The migrants' descendants learned to use microliths (tiny stone tools) and flourished, and they may have driven the earlier archaic humans to extinction. Since we are concerned about the origins of yoga, we will delve into events and developments in South Asia, which later developed into the nation-states of India, Pakistan, Afghanistan, Bangladesh, Sri Lanka, Bhutan, Nepal, Myanmar, and Maldives.

Based on the archaeological remains of long-gone communities and linguistic evidence, we know that South Asians are a mixture born out of four major prehistoric migrations between sixty-five thousand and 3,500 years ago. The first wave came from Africa, when a band of *Homo sapiens* made their way into the Indian subcontinent; these migrants are known as the First Indians.[3] The second wave (7000–1900 BCE) came from early Iranian farmers from the Zagros Mountains, who mixed with the First Indians and established the agriculture-centered urban Harappan civilization. The remains of the first farming settlement that grew wheat and barley is in a village called Mehrgarh in Baluchistan. This ancient urban settlement was a mighty one, with two centers in Harappa and Mohenjadaro, and the echoes of this ancient culture resonate in India even today. The third wave, who came from China, brought Austroasiatic languages to South-east Asia around 2000 BCE. This language family has two subfamilies, Munda and Khasi, which are spoken by people from modern Jharkhand in central India and Assam-Meghalaya in northeast India respectively.

The last wave (2000–1500 BCE) were herders, pastoral people from the central Asian steppes* who called themselves Aryan, a name with many connotations that emerge much later in human history. Genetic studies of human fossils from this period reveal a mixed ancestry of ancient Iranians, Anatolians (ancient Turkey), and Southeast Asian hunter-gatherers. The

---

* Regions encompassing ancient Iran or Persia, Turkmenistan, Uzbekistan, Kazakhstan, Afghanistan, and western Siberia.

Indo-Aryans—also called the Vedic people, as they were the primary composers of the Vedas—had a completely different culture, languages, and social structures, and they subsequently came to dominate most of north India. Below are some salient features of the most relevant threads to our study of yoga.

The Enigmatic Harappans

There is a bronze statue of a young girl with a rather cheeky hand on her hip, looking straight at us with a sassy gaze. Is she a dancer? Or is she merely striking a pose for the sculptor, much like artists' models do today? Next, there is a magnificent horned figure seated on a throne in a yoga-like pose, surrounded by an elephant, a tiger, a rhinoceros, a buffalo, and two deer. Is he a preeminent yogi? A divine figure who is the master of all of nature? Is it a goddess with an elaborate headdress? There are many hypotheses about the figures depicted on this seal, famously called the Pashu-pati (Lord of the Beasts), and arguments rage on about its significance in the annals of yoga history. Then there is a short statue of a bearded figure with eyes half closed, a nicely groomed beard, and thick lips. He has a decorative garment over his left shoulder and an ornament on his forehead; he is called the priest-king, someone with authority. Sculptures like this were common in the Harappan civilization (5500–1900 BCE).

The first archaeological site for Harappa, also known as the Indus Valley Civilization, was discovered in 1921. The land was fertile and conducive to experiments in agriculture, so nomadic peoples from Iran, Anatolia, and Turkmenistan settled into early crop-farming lifestyles and intermingled with the First Indians. The remains of the villages of this civilization are located in modern-day northwestern India, Baluchistan, and Pakistan. The excavations uncovered well-planned cities with baked brick houses, elaborate irrigation and sanitation systems, great baths, and clusters of uniformly spaced buildings. The Harappans thrived in a cosmopolitan society with trade exchanges between faraway lands such as Egypt and China. It was the most populated civilization among its contemporaries, spanning around 750,000 square miles.[4]

The material remains of the civilization bear no evidence of a powerful military. The weapons found are stone maces and clay pellets with axes and daggers. They do not seem fearsome or even well developed and may have been meant for ceremonies and rituals. There may have been an "internalization of customs, practices and regulations by the people through long habituation, in which temporal institutions assume the nature of an immutable cosmic order."[5] In other words, as there is no evidence of militaristic enforcement, the organized and yet benevolent towns point to an influential and insular theocracy consisting of priest-kings who were the religio-political heads who most likely lived or worked in towering citadels overlooking a vast terrace. The lack of a military in the presence of such homogeneity may be because of an emphasis of a collectivist culture that was informed by the theological heads of state, i.e., the priest-kings.

Even though there may not have been a monarchy, there is some evidence of stratification via a marked difference in the sizes of the homes. The poor had smaller homes, and the affluent had larger dwellings. There is also a marked uniformity of the layouts of urban centers in Harappan society, with very little variation; even the dimensions of bricks are alike. There are many seals that depict somber as well as raucous rituals and ceremonies, along with representations of *lingam* (phallus) and *yoni* (vulva). Both these symbols, along with those on the Pashu-pati seal (regarded as proto-Shiva),[6] are developed further in Shiva and goddess worship. There are many seals with one or two unicorns, buffalo-horned deities, multiple mother goddesses, bangles worn on wrists, and the peepal tree. Many elements of this time period still persist in South Asian culture a couple of thousand years later. For instance, some of the symbols and worship of the goddesses emerge from these times. The peepal tree is revered as a sacred plant even now, there are homes in villages in India constructed around a central courtyard, and bangles are still worn as adornments.

Some other seals depict chariots with solid wheels drawn by humped bulls. While many kinds of cattle, including cows, are present in the archaeological remains, the bull is given primal importance rather than the cow. This is an important clue about who the Harappans are *not*, rather than who they are, as we will see later.

The main script of this culture is yet undeciphered. Thus, much of their civilization, including their religion and politics, remain a great mystery; they are an enigma. Linguistic scholars agree, though, that the languages were proto-Dravidian, which is the source of Tamil, Telugu, Malayalam, Kannada, and Gondi, spoken by nearly a fifth of the population of modern India. Historians posit that there were many languages, as the civilization was vast, and the seals suggest that there was one standard script that was used throughout the region.[7] The most ancient languages in India are thus the Dravidian languages, rather than Sanskrit, as is commonly thought. One of the great mysteries of this period is: How did the proto-Dravidian languages of the Harappans, who lived in northwestern India, move across to the south—and most importantly, why?

There are many theories to illuminate how the Harappan/proto-Dravidian languages may have traveled to the south, including the old Tamil legend of the great Rishi Agastya's triumph over the proud Vindhya Mountains that separate the north from the south. The story goes that the Vindhya Mountains' colossal growth had even the mighty sun working hard. Thus Agastya, using all his *siddhis* (spiritual powers), commanded them to bow before him so he could cross them along with eighteen families of the Velir clan, and he asked them to not grow until he came back. He never returned and stayed on in the south, establishing the Tamil languages.

The Harappans were urbane, had well-planned civic amenities, and most likely did not have a monarch or a designated place of worship, as there are no remains of a temple or a palace. The possible reasons for the decline of the might of the Harappan cities are many. It may have been due to a long drought that resulted in large-scale deforestation, and environmental changes leading to an increase in disease; or it may have been due to great floods that are mentioned in later texts, such as the Shatapatha Brahmana.[8] These calamities, along with the foray of new warrior-like arrivals from the Central Asian steppes caused a dissolution of the civilization and the movement of peoples to the east and south, along with their cultural practices, beliefs, and languages. It is important to reiterate that this was a period when there was a great deal of merging together of different threads of migrant populations who settled and then spread out to different parts of ancient India, forming the complex and colorful tapestry we know today.

The Vedic Pastoralists

As the Harappan civilization disintegrated, pastoralists arrived from the steppes of Iran after traveling in search of greener pastures, literally, as they were a cattle-breeding community who cleared dense forests to settle into farming villages. They brought with them a group of Indo-European languages, early Sanskrit being one of them, and called themselves the Aryans, or the "nobles," and were organized into different tribes who gradually transitioned from their nomadic wanderings into an agrarian life. Agriculture led to land ownership and the appointment of a king as the protector of land and its resources.

It was during this time that the Rig Veda was composed. Anthropomorphic imagery emerges in the Rig Veda alongside elements of nature in a combination that shows an intimacy, an interdependence with and reverence for the phenomenal-material world. The Rig Veda consists of hymns praising the might of a pantheon of deities like Agni, the god of fire who was accorded a high status as the divine ruler of the sacrificial rituals (or *yajna*s) and who was also the deity of the domestic hearth. Thus, Agni bore witness to sacred ceremony and marriage rites. Varuna was the god of wind, and Indra, the king of all the Gods, as a ruler of thunder and rain was deemed to be of paramount stature in the Vedic pantheon (who resembles Zeus, the Greek god). Surya, the deity of the sun, was also revered as the goddess Gayatri.

There are a few goddesses, too, like Ushas, the goddess of dawn, bringing light and auspiciousness, dispelling darkness in all the realms, and associated with *rta*, cosmic and moral order. There is Prithvi, goddess of earth, described as stable, fertile, and nourishing all of creation; she has a male consort, Dyaus, deity of the sky. There is Aditi, the boundless, the free one, the benevolent mother of kings and gods alike. She is often identified as a divine cow, perhaps in homage to the most important animal for a pastoral community; her milk is described as *soma*, the sacred elixir. The gendered roles are evident in the gods' attributes: The goddesses mostly are benign and nourishing, maternal, almost always with a male consort. The hymns are eulogies, propitiating to earn the benediction of the deities, the gods and goddesses who need to be appeased for blessings of health, fertility, rain, and protection from enemies. In one hymn Aditi is asked to free a petitioner who is tied up like a thief.[9]

The *yajna*s and other Vedic rituals also necessitated a command of language where words and speech had to be precise. The blessings from Vak, the goddess of speech and words, were summoned for the creation of esoteric mantras and poetic metaphors equating the cascade of the river Saraswati to the fluency of one's language. In the later Vedic Age, the deity Vak became Saraswati, worshiped by millions of Hindus today as a deity of learning. Additionally, *yajna*s necessitated precise calculations of planetary positions and proficiency in mathematics; thus there was a burgeoning of sophisticated scholarship in astrology, astronomy, and Vedic mathematics. The Vedas also explored profound philosophical and metaphysical questions regarding the creation of the cosmos, the nature of eternal consciousness, and the possibilities of life after death and reincarnation.

There was a genuine veneration of and a pragmatic relationship with the cow, as Indo-Aryans were primarily cattle breeders. Rituals and sacrifices were considered necessary for summoning blessings from the sky-dwelling gods who presided over nature, and these could be only conducted by the Brahmins, which compounded their position of power. Beef meat, mostly from the castrated steers, was eaten on special occasions and was part of ritualistic offerings during sacrifices to deities. The Gopatha Brahmana from the Atharva Veda refers to animal killings. A bull (*vrsabha*) was sacrificed to Indra, a dappled cow to the Maruts (gods of storm and lightning), and a copper-colored cow to the Asvins, the twin deities of medicine and health. "The *aganyadheya*, which was a preparatory rite preceding all public sacrifices, required a cow to be killed."[10] The cow was valuable property that conferred social status and economic currency, and it was considered an exalted animal, to be protected against cattle raids from rival tribes. The reverence for the cow of the Vedic period thus did not exclude consumption of the meat as a sacrificial offering. One of the many reasons why the theory that the Vedic people are the same as the Harappans (and thus the original inhabitants) is debunked is because of the relevance given to the bull in the Harappan civilization (not the cow) and to the cow in the Vedic civilization (not the bull).

Around 500 BCE, the renunciate ascetics known as sramanas withdrew from a stratified Vedic tradition. They lived either in the forests or on the outskirts and challenged some of the claims of the Vedas, including the necessity of sacrificial rituals. People practiced asceticism to achieve one of two goals: either the procurement of magical and mystical powers by practicing austerities and meditation, or the renouncement of the demands of an increasingly complex and violent society. The sramanas, moved by the brutality, passionately advocated for ahimsa (nonviolence or nonharming) toward all beings, and they were fiercely critical of the Vedic rituals that included animal sacrifice. They preached against *himsa*, violence against all beings. Ahimsa, one of the most fundamental concepts and principles of yoga, was thus born as a repudiation of violence against animals and brutal competition between groups.

While some sramanas retreated to forests to delve into the meaning of life beyond this material world, some of them came back to challenge the casteist society that later coalesced to birth Buddhism and Jainism. Vegetarianism was integrated into Brahmanism around 600 BCE to counter the growing popularity of Buddhism and Jainism, the more egalitarian traditions that welcomed folks from all classes and castes. These two sramanic traditions also influenced the development of the tenets of Advaita Vedanta (non-dualism), which emphasized the seamless continuum of the microcosm and macrocosm. However, there were ontological differences, too. While Advaita Vedanta conceptualizes all matter, every human being, and every non-human being as Atma, a manifestation of the supreme Param-atma, Buddha preached about *anatta* (the Pali word for no-Self), the teaching that the perennial notion of selfhood refers to something that does not exist.

Vegetarianism became an integral teaching in many later Brahmanic texts. However, not all Brahmins are vegetarians. For instance, I come from the Konkani-speaking Gaud Saraswat caste, from modern Goa and the coastal Karnataka region, where fish is considered as a part of the diet; thus there are pescatarian Brahmins too. Kashmiri pandits also eat meat, except for pork.

Today, vegetarianism is seen as a symbol of the "communal identity of all Hindus and obscurantist and fundamentalist forces who refuse to appreciate that the cow and the bull were important in a myriad ways in the Vedic and subsequent Brahmanic and non-Brahmanical traditions. Meat was quite often a part of haute cuisine in ancient India,"[11] as D. N. Jha asserts in the book *The Myth of the Holy Cow*. Beef, a part of the diets of Muslims, Christians, and Dalits, is a significant factor for discrimination and violence today, with the rise of *gau-rakshak* (cow protector) militia-like groups whipping up public frenzy over "anti-Hindu culture." Jha writes about the pressure and threats he experienced from right-wing politicians during the publishing of his book in 2001. According to Human Rights Watch, "between May 2015 and December 2018, at least 44 people—36 of them Muslims—were killed across 12 Indian states. Over that same period, around 280 people were injured in over 100 different incidents across 20 states" in attacks "led by so-called cow protection groups."[12] This is deeply ironic because the Vedas, considered to be the quintessential text of the people who were later called Hindus, include hundreds of verses dedicated to elaborate descriptions of sacrifices of cows and other animals.

The Emergence of Jaati

In a late hymn of the Rig Veda called the Purusa Sukhtam, there is an allegorical reference to the genesis of caste:

> *When they divided the Man, into how many parts did they divide him?*
> *What was his mouth, what were his arms, what were his thighs and his feet called?*
> *The brahman was his mouth, of his arms were made the warrior.*
> *His thighs became the vaishya, of his feet the shudra was born.*
> *With Sacrifice the gods sacrificed to Sacrifice, these were the first of the sacred laws.*
> *These mighty beings reached the sky, where are the eternal spirits, the gods.*[13]

In this verse, "Man" refers to *purusa*, universal consciousness or the cosmic being. The different limbs denote different occupations, offering a glimpse into the early stratifications in Vedic society. From a textual standpoint, the genesis of varna, a framework of social stratification based on occupation and class, can be traced back to these verses. This is the foundational myth of the Brahmin class, establishing social hierarchies, and it is from an earlier layer of the Rig Veda.[14] Many scholars assert, however, that these verses were a later addition to the text and were inserted to impart a divine sanctity and legitimacy to the varna system.

When they first came to India, the Indo-Aryans were organized into three classes (varnas) based on occupation: the warriors, the priests, and everyone else. This was not a hereditary designation, nor were there rules for intermarriages between the classes. The movement toward the development of a hereditary system began when the Indo-Aryans encountered the Indigenous, darker-skinned Dasas (the First Indians), who worshipped different gods and spoke different languages.[15] The color distinction not only provides an important insight into the development of the varnas (a Sanskrit word for "color") but also is a harbinger of the color prejudice that persists today. These clashes between the new arrivals and the indigenous Dasas became a part of the stories in the Puranas, the Mahabharata, and the Ramayana, where the lighter-skinned Indo-Aryans are depicted as celestial beings or devas and gods, and the darker-skinned Dasas as fierce and aggressive *rakshasa*s. Any people who were not from the Aryan tribes were called *mleccha*, or barbarians. These included forest dwellers and people south of the Vindhyas who were regarded as subhuman, malformed, or hideous-looking *rakshasa*s.[16]

Over centuries, the varna framework developed four categories: Brahmins (scholars/priests), Kshatriyas (warriors), Vaishyas (traders/merchants) and Shudras (farmers/artisans). The former three categories were considered to be savarna (in the varnas) *dvija*, or twice-born: The first birth is biological, and the second is a ritualistic initiation into education or apprenticeship according to varna status. The Shudras who provided the labor for the Brahmins, Kshatriyas, and Vaishyas were excluded from initiation rituals. There was a fifth category, the *avarna*s, heterogeneous groups of people whose identities were complex. They were the Indigenous tribes of South Asia (Adivasis), also called the Dasas. Avarnas were also people of mixed Vedic-Dasa origin and worked as menial laborers (later called Dalit/Bahujan). Even today the word Dasa translates to servant or slave. To ensure ease and accessibility for the reader, I will mostly use the terms savarna, avarna, and caste as umbrella terms, unless the narrative requires further details on the specific elements of these labels.

In the beginning, there was relative fluidity between the four varna categories, and status was not entirely fixed, even though the Brahmins and the Kshatriyas vied for social-political dominance. However, by the later Vedic Age (1100–500 BCE), ritual-oriented Brahmanism was the dominant religion of the elite. "Vedic" Sanskrit was the language of religion and politics, as the medium both for elaborate rituals and for documents of the state. The language in this form was zealously guarded by the Brahmins. Prakrit, a more vernacular variation of Sanskrit, had many regional influences, such as Magadhi, Maharashtri, Gandhari, Pali, and Shauraseni.

The urbanization of society, coupled with trade and commerce between people and the proliferation of artisan guilds (*shreni*), meant that newer power dynamics emerged. Each guild lived in a specific section of town, so that members of a guild lived and worked together and thus had such a "closeknit relationship that they came to be regarded as a sub-caste."[17] As villages formed, land cultivated, and trade expanded, the work that was needed to create, sustain, and protect property and wealth got more defined. The tribal kingdoms were made up of villages, with the family or the clan as the nucleus. A king was appointed to govern as a ruling authority with checks and balances from the tribal assemblies, and his role later was accorded divine status. The people who owned agricultural land and traded produce and products became wealthier and thus more influential, which sometimes gave them pathways to upward mobility in the varna stratification system. For instance, the founder of the Nanda dynasty, Mahapadma Nanda (400–340 BCE), was the son of a Shudra mother.[18]

This verse from the Rig Veda is another indication that occupations were not entirely rigid or based solely on birth:

> *I am a poet; my dad's a physician*
> *and Mom a miller with grinding stones.*
> *With diverse thoughts we all strive for wealth,*
> *going after it like cattle.*[19]

This was also the atmosphere that produced the political doctrine *matsya-nyaya*: "unbridled competition in which the powerful preyed upon the weak, or to use the language of the texts, 'where the big fish swallowed the little fish.'"[20] The last line in the verse above, "going after it like cattle," is important as it refers to rivalry and contentiousness between groups.

As migrations into ancient India continued, each new group became a subcaste as they assimilated into the larger varna structure. The intermingling of these groups gave rise to hundreds of jaatis. *Jaati* (or "birth") refers to an endogamous unit within which one must marry. Members of a jaati are part of a descent group, traditionally assigned to a specific occupation. Each jaati has its own traditions, with unique cuisines, dialects, rituals, traditions, symbols, dress codes, and art forms. The emergence and development of the jaatis as a rigid marker of one's identity took place over hundreds of years as occupations became hereditary, i.e., a son of a Brahmin became a Brahmin, a soldier's son became a soldier, and so on, not by choice of occupation or inclination but by birth alone. Endogamy ossified one's dharma or one's role in society, with diminishing access to material and spiritual resources. It became the norm that one had to marry within the jaati, so the jaati system became more rigid as it allowed very little upward mobility in the hierarchy. This was and continues to be harmful and violent for the ones who are at the receiving end of this of power structure: the Shudras, the Dalit folks, and the Bahujan.

As Brahmanism spread through the region, there was an absorption of ideas, resources, and practices from diverse cultures and traditions, including appropriating deities and beliefs from the non–Indo-Aryan (those later called Adivasis, Bahujan, and Dalits). Although the earliest portions of the Vedas appear to be relatively free from the influence of Indigenous cultures, the impact of these cultures becomes increasingly evident in the later portions of the Vedas.[21] This means that there was an increase in encounters and intermingling between the Indo-Aryans and non–Indo-Aryans. Not all of these encounters were peaceful, and many of these confrontations were encapsulated in *itihasa* literature as conflicts between the Devas and the Rakshasas.

The hierarchies of varna-jaatis persisted in every realm, not just the abstract, esoteric dimension of spiritual emancipation but also—and perhaps most importantly—extending to resources like land, education, employment, and housing. While the Kshatriyas exercised material control through land ownership, Brahmin men exerted a monopoly over intellectual and spiritual knowledge. There is a substantial and "profound inequality between the castes in terms of productive resources, social status and access to knowledge."[22] The construction of subservient classes also guaranteed bonded labor for the savarnas. The avarnas were made to do the labor that was considered menial, such as removal of human waste, cremation, and working with leather and meat. Though the tasks were integral for the socioeconomic functioning of the community, the people who performed the labor were considered to be polluting. From this came the terrible concept of untouchability, which gradually became entrenched into all dimensions of society. These oppressive hierarchies were legitimized through philosophical and religious texts, establishing a continuum of religion-culture-politics-economics.

Dr. Bhimrao Ambedkar, a revolutionary Dalit leader and the author of the Indian constitution, makes this eloquent statement in his seminal book *Annihilation of Caste*: "Caste system is not merely a division of labor. It is also a division of laborers. Civilized society undoubtedly needs division of labor. But in no civilized society is division of labor accompanied by this unnatural division of laborers into watertight compartments. The caste system is a hierarchy in which the divisions of laborers are graded one above the other."[23] The gradual establishment of Brahmanism—a term preferred by the caste abolitionist movement, as it points to the earliest form of religion rather than to Hinduism (a term that evolved much later)—creates what Thenmozhi Soundararajan, founder of Equality Labs and author of *The Trauma of Caste*, refers to as a "dominator system of caste apartheid . . . an animating ideology that justifies the dehumanization and destruction of caste-oppressed peoples."[24]

Around 600 BCE, people settled into specific geographical regions. There emerged a need to organize and identify boundaries and methods for administration, giving rise to republics made up of one or many tribes and monarchies. The republics were composed of either a single tribe or a confederacy of multiple tribes such as the Vrijis and Yadavas, and were some of the earliest democracies known to humanity. While scholars differ on the administrative details of the republics, most agree that governmental decision-making involved "the meeting of the representatives of tribes or the heads of families"[25] and was grounded on the idea that sovereignty rested in the hands of the people, not a king. The republican-oriented tribes were far more welcoming of disruptive, heterodox thought, and so it is not surprising that two very influential thought leaders would be birthed in this ethos of individual thought: Gautam Buddha from the Shakya tribe, and Mahavira, the preeminent teacher of Jainism, from the Jnatrika tribe.

Around the same time, the early Upanishads were composed by renunciants who were within and on the margins of the Vedic traditions, ascetics referred to as the *vratyas* in the Rig Veda. Upanishad means "sitting near," and the term refers to the connections between concepts, or it can suggest disciples sitting near a teacher. These mystics lived deep in the forests or outside the bustling village-towns. The Upanishads offered a poetic distillation of the spiritual inquiries of the Vedas and added to them a synthesis of sorts of Vedic and sramanic thought in a more conversational Sanskrit form, making it accessible to more seekers. As Buddhism and Jainism grew in influence, there was a synergetic exchange that contributed to philosophical inquiries into the purpose and meaning of life. In contrast to the Vedas, which emphasized discipline in rituals, the Upanishadic teachings were concerned with inquiries into transmigration of spirit, samsara, karma, and the nature of consciousness, and they emphasized discipline of mind and body, or *yoga*. Thus, the earliest form of yoga was borne from a crystallization of these sramanic and Upanishadic streams of thought.

By 700 BCE, monarchies were replacing tribal communities, with escalating tensions within and between rival clans, giving rise to many struggles for power.[26] The conflicts between Buddhists and Brahmins in particular were bitter and violent, as each sought a place on the altar and the throne. Buddhists accepted people from all backgrounds, and in sharp contrast to Brahminism, unequivocally rejected caste. Buddhist texts depict members of the Chandala—the caste who worked in cremation grounds, who were considered to be untouchable—in pivotal roles. In addition, the Vaselasutta—a part of the Sutta Nippata, a Buddhist text in Pali—describes the ancient hero Matanga as the one who is revered by nobles and Brahmins alike.

The Buddhist ideals for society and the role of state were far more egalitarian. There were expectations from a ruler: to be a righteous *cakkavati* ("king" in Pali) who followed the "wheel of *dhamma*—providing salaries to bureaucrats, capital to merchants, seed to farmers and help to the poor."[27] The conceptualization and practice of sangha was integral, "since it was the realm where meditation was practiced and enlightenment was sought, rather than ritualism, what was encouraged was righteous relationships."[28] The Buddhist emphasis on simplicity, nonviolence, and nonattachment was a sharp contrast to and a criticism of Brahmanism, which centered on elaborate offerings and stratified relationships within the varna system. However, this aspiration to egalitarianism did not extend to equality across genders. Buddhists did to some degree accept women as nuns, especially during the time of the Buddha, but Jainism was far more restrictive, with women aspirants having to work harder to neutralize the accrual of karma. Almost all the prevalent faith and spiritual traditions had texts or teachings that conceptualized women as spiritual impediments who were also physically incapable of attaining salvation due to the stigma associated with menstruation. (This idea will be explored more in the next chapter.)

While Brahmanism flourished in the urban centers, people from the rural areas and the forest and mountain dwellers lived with "their ears close to the earth, who whispered to them her secrets as long as they did not wound her breasts with the plough."[29] Some of these rituals of deep connection to the mysteries of nature—worship of village gods or *grama devatas*, myths of creation and destruction, sacred rituals of obeisance to the earth goddesses, with a primary concern for fertility—were co-opted, integrated, and appropriated as the Vedic people spread out into the forests. Thus there is an underlying tension between region-specific tribal traditions and the Brahmanical orthodox traditions. This tension will be explored further in chapter 3.

As forests were cleared and people settled into agriculture-oriented societies, Vedic society became increasingly patriarchal. The woman's role was in relationship to the men in her life as a dutiful daughter or daughter-in-law, as a supporter of her husband or father, and as a birther of sons to continue the lineage. Her piety, loyalty, and chastity was her dharma.

Vedic Literature and Brahmanism

Brahmanical orthodoxy regards a few texts as essential to the tradition. There are four main classes or genres of Vedic literature that emerge in more or less chronological order (during approximately 1500–800 BCE): the Vedic Samhitas, the Brahmanas, the Aranyakas, and the Upanishads. Each Vedic Samhita has its own school and its own Brahmana (not to be confused with Brahmin, the scholar), Aranyaka, and Upanishad. The Vedic Samhitas are largely Indo-Aryan in origin, and much of their content was probably brought into the Indic region by the Indo-European tribes.[30] The four Vedic Samhitas are Rig, Yajur, Sama, and Atharva. In addition to these compositions are the Dharmashastras (legal codes), epics (the Mahabharata and the Ramayana), the Darshanas (philosophical systems), and the Puranas (mythological compositions).

Another issue related to the Vedic texts that is of primary importance to us, as investigators of Brahmanical orthodoxy, is intertextuality, because it explains the relationship between the Vedas and texts such as the Dharmashastras, the epic literature, and the Puranas. Intertextuality is "the repetition from text to text of unarticulated yet formative rules and regulations that determine the general nature of language and textuality in a given tradition."[31] Vedic tenets infused the ethos, culture, and politics of many South Asian countries. The doctrines of rebirth, karma, and dharma put forth in the Vedas were enacted in the Mahabharata and Ramayana and were reinforced in the legal texts and the Puranas. While most people in modern India do not know the esoteric content of the Vedas, most savarna people consider the Vedas with great reverence and even worship them as the divine.

Much of the epic literature and the Puranas was translated into regional languages and thus was influenced by the worldviews of regional scholars and sages. This also meant that the authority of the Vedas and other Vedic literature and the Brahmin authors came to define the dominant philosophical and spiritual narratives in the region.

Vedic tenets recommended a particular life sequence for the savarna. The *ashramas*, or stages in the savarna man's life, were student (*brahmachari*), householder (*grhsta*), elder withdrawing from social life into the forest (*vanaprastha*), and finally ascetic (*sanyasi*). These stages were not for women, but women were important in upholding the sequence. In the *grhsta* (householder) stage, one had to marry. Wives were an integral part of many rituals as participants. The addition of the *sanyasi* ashrama was a response to the growing influence of the sramanas, a way to include the more esoteric pursuits of human aspiration. This philosophical framework guides the savarnas, an undergirding of sorts for all actions, activities, and endeavors for one's lifetime. It also established the savarna man, especially the Brahmin, as the primary curator and conduit of spiritual and liberatory knowledge and praxis.

Many of the concepts in Vedic literature are used to establish a legitimacy and a mystical sanctity for class and caste hierarchies. For instance, the two foundational principles of karma (action) and dharma (order or obligation, or it can also be loosely translated as religion) started out in context of the Vedic rituals and bore no ethical, legal, or larger social significance. They referred to a right way to conduct the *yajna*s, as the sacrificial rituals formed the focus of religious life. Through time, these concepts took on social and ethical dimensions. The principle of karma operated in conjunction with the idea that spirit (Atma) is eternal and that even though the physical body expires, it is reincarnated again and again in cycles of birth and death. According to this idea, one's quality of life, including the caste one is born into, is based on the virtues or vileness of one's past lives' karmas. If one fulfilled their societal duties well and did not stray from their varna, then they accumulated *punya* (virtues) and may even go toward the path of moksha (liberation from the cycle of birth and death). The parameters of right conduct were governed by the varna and later the jaati that one was born into, rather than personal agency (with a few exceptions, which will be explored later in this book). If one flouted the rules of the varna one was born into, either by marrying someone outside the jaati or by socializing with them (even through touch), then the consequence was punishment of some sort during this life or rebirth as avarna or an animal in the next life.

The law texts—such as the Manava Dharmashastra, written sometime around the first century CE—expounded upon each person's positionality in the upholding of the social order (dharma) and in connection with universal order (*rta*). The rigidity of the jaati system developed gradually through prohibition of intermarriage between the groups and was observed to preserve the "purity" of lineage, thus maintaining resources and privileges accorded to the savarna. While the Manava Dharmashastra (more commonly known as the Manu Smriti) upheld the duties, rituals, and class and caste structures of the Vedic people, it was not a book of overarching law that was used for governance until British colonialism, which will be discussed more in the next chapter.

The Vedas, the Upanishads, the Puranas, and the Dharmashastras were "self-referential," ensuring a "self-conscious adaptation of literary structures and devices found in one text or textual tradition by another text or tradition."[32] This reflexivity or intertextuality also meant an amplification of a particular worldview—that of Brahmin men. The orality of the compositions also meant there was a porosity and permeability, allowing an absorption of non-Vedic elements as well as a diffusion from the Vedic ideals into the margins of the community. The Rig Veda was preserved orally for centuries, even when writing was used, with an emphasis on precision of narration, enunciation, and memorization of its 1,028 poems.[33] They were deemed as *shruthi*, that which is heard, not only because they were considered to be transmitted through a sacred conduit as blessings from the gods and/or spiritually realized beings, but also because these were oral teachings from teacher (guru) to disciple (*shishya*) through a lineage from one to the other (*parampara*). Even though the Puranic compositions offer homage to the central tenets of the Vedic teachings, they differ on the forms, places, and deities of worship. Temples and home altars became the norm. Each caste and sect had its own norm and tradition. There were reimaginations and reinterpretations of the epics and the Puranas, with layers of meaning accumulating over centuries.

Most scholars believe that the Mahabharata, for instance, was composed over a period of eight hundred years. Thus, there were additions, editions, and tweaks that were reflections of what was deemed important in that particular period in a particular region. Ramayana, composed by Valmiki, is an epic poem (*maha kaavya*) that is a part of *itihasa* literature. It is considered as one of the two most important chronicles of the Indic region centering around the kingdom of Kosala (the modern Indian state of Uttar Pradesh), along with the Mahabharata. As in most oral traditions, the Ramayana has earlier and later layers, with embellishments that have accreted around a "core element of truth."[34] The dates span from 500 BCE for the early layers to 500 CE for the later ones.

Even though the language of composition for both the epics was Sanskrit, once they got written down, they were recorded in diverse scripts, including Sharada, Mewari, Maithili, Bengali, Telugu, Kannada, Nandinagari, Grantha, and Malayalam. This is a critical point that is often overlooked. The heterogeneity of languages assured a plurality of worldviews, a multiplicity in the cultural representations and characterizations of a story. The texts were translated through varying lived experiences and media. This elasticity made the stories stay alive, expressed and enacted through stone, drama, and song, in every language and dialect, taking in the distinctive flavors of each region. Therefore, it is important for us to consider and study the history of a text, how the teachings were used or misused, and the positionalities of the folks whose translations we are studying in order to unravel the embedded social contexts. We need to excavate the impact of the texts in all facets, the political and the spiritual, because these texts are often used as cornerstones of values and the foundations of dominant cultures. We will explore this further in chapter 4 in the story of Radha and Krishna.

As discerning yoga practitioners, there is a need for us to tease out the elements of oppression and understand the historical contexts so we can get to the liberatory truths. Thus, we study not only concepts, tenets, and practices in yogic texts but also how they shape and have shaped caste and gender dynamics. The texts are situated in the sociocultural ethos of the time of their composition, and they have been operationalized for maintaining systemic and structural hierarchies. By conferring legitimacy upon the texts as "tradition," there is a validation of the essentiality of caste and a mythologizing of the subjugation of peoples outside the varna system. There also have been movements and moments of defiance through history, especially on the part of those who were harmed and marginalized. Some of the more consequential ones, like the Bhakti movement, are known, while others have been quieter microrebellions that are startling in their resilience in the face of overwhelming odds. These are the voices we can heed today to ignite and nourish our own forms of embodied resistance.

2

IS YOGA HINDU?

We begin by asking perhaps one of the most contested questions: Is yoga Hindu? And this leads us to two other questions: Who are the Hindus? What is yoga? This chapter delves into these two big questions. Both of them are salient queries that are particularly in need of clarification given the broad brushstrokes of a forged uniformity that defines "Indian culture" as a Hindu culture. Uniformity is conducive to ease of governance, and it limits the possibility of challenging paradoxes and deviations of diverse thought, lived experiences, and values. Yoga is not a one-size-fits-all practice; nor does it come from one particular religion or culture. Rather, it evolved and is situated in a plethora of traditions, religions, and regions, and yet most practitioners would find it challenging to tease out these integrated threads.

An internet search on the word *yoga* reveals that most people associate it with fitness and health. Some may refer to its psychosomatic benefits, or what is ubiquitously known as "mental health" and "stress reduction." Most do not know that the physical asana practice has a history, or that "it" is a composite of numerous traditions interspersed with post-nineteenth-century health- and fitness-oriented modalities. Thus, transnational modern yoga is an overlay of modern and ancient insight into the body and mind. While some curious practitioners or yoga teacher training curricula may include excerpts from Patanjali's sutras, *Hatha Yoga Pradipika*, the Puranas, the Upanishads, or the Gita, there is less awareness of the differences and overlaps in these philosophies. The threads of caste are invisible in this complex, colorful, multihued yogic tapestry.

One Instagram post boldly said that Chaturanga is also known as "Hindu push-ups."[1] Thousands responded enthusiastically to this claim. There are many asanas that have the names of deities like Ananta, Hanuman, or Devi, so it is understandable how yoga and Hinduism can be conflated. The dominant narrative both in India and in the West is that yoga has Hindu roots. Based on this notion, many yoga studios often set up idols of deities like Ganesha; chant *stotra*s in praise of Shiva, Vishnu, or Devi; and celebrate festivals like Diwali, Holi, and Navratri, with an understanding that all is within the realm of yoga. This bolsters the aspects of one path of "yoga," but certainly not all. These conflations and overlaps of yoga and Hinduism can advance the communal ideologies of the Hindu right and/ or reinforce the Western conservative notion that yoga is an exotic, heathen tradition that is unfit for secular education or for folks from different religions. Thus, it is important for us as discerning practitioners to know how to locate the practices in geographic, social, and political contexts and examine the veracity of such claims.

The teachings of yoga evolved prior to the geopolitical formation of the nation-state of India. Some of (what are considered) the core texts of yoga were composed before the label of "Hindu" was applied to a wide array of traditions. The previous chapter laid the foundations for the identities of the people who developed the technologies of yoga. This chapter will deconstruct some of the paradoxes of both yoga and Hinduism. We will delve into the most well-known traditions or texts so they can serve as a map for the journey of an avid yoga practitioner. To enumerate every single facet of yoga history is beyond the scope of this book or my own expertise; rather, the objective is to open a window for deeper, more comprehensive study.

To define the multidimensionality of Hinduism, I will use a beloved dish of the land, the ubiquitously known—and most misunderstood—dish that India is best known for: the curry. Contrary to the Western notion, curry spice is not made from "curry powder"; nor is there consensus for what goes into a curry. There is a curry made with every combination of every ingredient in India. Every home in India, every state, and every region within that state makes a different version with the same ingredients. Curries are veritable alchemies of fragrant spices and herbs, made with all kinds of lentils, meats, vegetables, and fruits in a wide array of combinations and bases. From coconut to *kokum* (a fruit), from lamb to *raajma*, from pungent mustard to sweet mangoes, we make thousands of curries. Curries are culinary expressions of cultural, philosophical, regional, geographic, and social diversities.

Hinduism is like a curry. There are different expressions of what Hinduism means, how it is lived and experienced. For every "rule" in the Hindu system, there is a contradiction and a paradox; there are no absolutes. It is easier to define Hinduism by what it is not, rather than what it is. It is not a monolith; it is not a religion centered around a set of universally observed practices, a central canon, or even common ideas about life. A Hindu can be atheist, agnostic, or polytheistic. There is a place for the sublime, the mundane, the violent, and the gross. There is an embrace of both elaborate ritual (*shastra vidhi*) and ascetic frugality. Every idea is examined and debated. There is an emphasis on right action (dharma) rather than right doctrine. Orthopraxy is more important than orthodoxy. Although there may not be a wholehearted embrace of contradictions and paradoxes at all times among all Hindus, there is some understanding of some paradoxes for some of the time in Indic history. There is a dire need to reclaim the complexity and heterogeneity of thought, perspectives, and lived experiences in resistance to deliberate and strategic erasure by dominant cultures everywhere.

The word *Hindu* itself is not from the land it is mostly associated with. It has its etymological roots in Old Persian (fourth century CE) and the term *al-hind* (in Arabic texts) encompassed all the people who lived on the other side of the River Sindhu, or the Indus River. Thus, it began as a geographical identification rather than a religious one that included diverse, heterogeneous belief systems and traditions. "Hindu" was thus a geopolitical identification that did not have a cogent religious connotation; nor did the people of the region self-identify as one until many centuries later, first with the arrival of the Muslims and then the Europeans. The word Hindu was never used in compositions such as the Vedas, the Puranas, the Bhagavad Gita, or the Upanishads; nor were these texts considered to be of significance to all Hindus. People used other identifiers, such as their caste, their region, or even the language they spoke. For example, I would say that I am a Gaud Saraswat Brahmin who speaks Konkani (a dialect) from Bangalore.

But before that, we get information from texts that indicate a more generalized meaning of the word. The first-century law book Manava Dharmashastra (Manu Smriti) does not use the word *Hindu* but does offer a geographical definition of the people to whom Manu's explication of dharma applies: "From the eastern sea to the western sea [the Indian Ocean and the Bay of the Bengal], the area in between the two mountains [the Himalayas and the Vindhyas] is what wise men call the Land of the Aryans. Where the black antelope ranges by nature, that should be known as the country fit for sacrifices; and beyond it is the country of the barbarians. The twice-born should make every effort to settle in these countries" (2.22–24).[2]

The verses above specify a location and adds qualifiers that reveal Manu's positionality. He describes a "country fit for sacrifices" and a "country of the barbarians," referring to the Vedic rituals of the Indo-Aryan people, and he asserts that those who do not belong there are the savage other. Over time many of these caste-aggrandizing themes steadily gain momentum and converge to impose a homogenous religious identity, as we will explore in this chapter.

There are a billion Hindus, but there is not one singular version of Hinduism that all members consider as the absolute truth. So who is a Hindu? Is there such a thing as "Hinduism"? To return to the metaphor of the curry, it has several ingredients in different combinations and permutations, and each family puts these together in their own unique way. Some of the ingredients of Hinduism are the concept of divinity, Atma, reincarnation, a pantheon of deities, different paths to moksha, four varnas, four ashramas, dharma, four Vedas, eighteen Puranas, law books, and expositions on astronomy and astrology. However, there is not one single set of doctrines that all Hindus agree with, that all Hindus consider as significant, or that are essentially and uniquely Hindu, because many were developed in conjunction with or as a response to other traditions.

Indic thought includes two important concepts—*astika*s and *nastika*s—that are contradictions of each other. *Astika*s, from the Sanskrit word *asti* meaning "there is," are people who accept the teachings of the Vedas regarding the interplay of Atma (individual consciousness) and Brahman (universal consciousness). *Nastika*s are inherently heterodox, people who doubt the veracity of teachings of the Vedas, the notion of a personal god, and the concept of the Self. They reject not only the esoteric philosophies and deities but also the stratified systems and regulatory laws created in the name of the deities. They accept people from all castes and clans and are thus more egalitarian in their ideals. The *nastika*s, such as Buddhists and Jains, also developed unique religious traditions outside the umbrella term of *Hindu*.

Even within the *astika*s there is a wide array of *darshana*s or perspectives that delve into different aspects of metaphysical, epistemological (theories of knowing), or soteriological (paths to salvation) issues. There are six major *astika* schools of philosophy, each offering unique and sometimes contrasting perspectives: Nyaya (logic), Vaisheshika (atomist or naturalist), Samkhya (dualistic principles of matter and consciousness), Mimamsa (critical investigation of the Vedas), Vedanta (encompassing the philosophies of the Vedas, e.g., the Upanishads), and, most relevant to our discussions, Yoga (praxis cultivating mind-body discipline for Self-realization, where Self is the Atma of Vedanta teachings or the Purusa of Samkhya).

Theism was also diverse. Vedic gods and goddesses were appeased through elaborate fire rituals (*yajna*s). The Puranas developed the idea of personal gods and expanded the mythologies of Shiva, Devi, and Vishnu. Puranic conceptualization of the divine appealed to everyday people for many reasons. A personal god or goddess, someone with the physical form of a deity, someone who could be addressed in prayers, an embodiment of the sacred, was more appealing to the human imagination than an abstraction of universal consciousness. Thus, most who are theistic may refer to bhakti (devotion) as a primary connection to their religion.

Bhakti is practiced in many ways: at an altar or in a space at home, or during a visit to the temple for *darshan* or *pooja* with symbolic, ritualistic offerings of prayer including mantras, flowers, fire, and incense. Hinduism is therefore a synthesis, a hybrid, syncretic in its many originations. It is an amalgamation of various philosophies, cultural elements, and ideologies, not a singular doctrine-oriented religion.

Although all those grouped under the mantle of Hinduism are vastly different, the scaffolding that has held such varied people together is varna-ashrama and subsequent development of the jaati system. Caste emerged as an economic-political and cultural fulcrum around which society was organized. As other religions came to the region and were integrated into the fabric through either voluntary or forced conversions, caste identity persisted. Thus, although one may be a Krishna-worshiping Vaishnava, or a Devi-worshiping Shakta, or both, or neither; although one may be a Muslim, a Christian, a Sikh, an atheist or an agnostic, caste was and is the common denominator undergirding all other identities.

Dr. Bhimrao Ambedkar articulates it thus: "The first and foremost thing that must be recognized is that Hindu society is a myth. The name Hindu is itself a foreign name. Hindu society as such does not exist. It is only a collection of castes. Each caste is conscious of its existence. Its survival is the be-all and end-all of its existence."[3]

Depending on one's lived experience, the porosity of the Hindu system (or Hinduism) is seen either as a positive, affirming aspect or as a violent overtaking of another's religion/belief system and practices. Dr. Sarvepalli Radhakrishnan, a Brahmin scholar and the second president of India, said that Hinduism is a belief "that truth was many-sided and different views contained different aspects of truth which no one could fully express."[4] Both of these viewpoints of Hinduism are rooted in contrasting lived experiences. To the ones oppressed by the caste system for nearly three thousand years, the caste system is synonymous with the Hindu, so there is a rejection of this label entirely. Hindu is an umbrella term encompassing different things for different people, and the centrality of caste cannot be denied or ignored because it is one of the only aspects that persist in almost every sect and tradition within that label, as well as in other religions in South Asia. Thus, deconstruction of caste history as well as a persistent unraveling of how it manifests in all the realms, including yoga, is imperative to cultivate spaces of healing that welcome everyone from all lived experiences.

Dharma: The Principal Ingredient

If there is one quintessential principle that can be named as a salient or principal ingredient in the Hindu curry, it would be dharma, which has a long, convoluted history. It is important for us to know the context of its evolution, as the word is used almost ubiquitously in yoga spaces and yet is little understood. It would not be hyperbolic to say that dharma is one of the fundamental principles that has shaped the socioreligious lives of not only Hindus but also Buddhists, Jains, and Sikhs. There is no word that is equivalent to *dharma* in the English language, which is one reason why it's a difficult word to translate. But that is not the only reason why. It is also because the meaning and the usage of the word has adapted to the shifting sands of time.

Dharma comes from the Sanskrit root word *dhr*, which means "to uphold or maintain" and is linked to *dharana*, which means "supporting." In this context it is related to the Vedic concept of cosmic order, *rta*. The Rig Veda expounds on dharma, as it is mentioned over sixty times in elaborations on rituals and duties that maintain the social order as a continuum of the natural and the heavenly domains of creation. Thus, from a Vedic perspective, dharma is a "commitment to holding apart heaven and earth, as well as other things such as plants, rivers and the four main castes in society."[5]

During the Vedic period, the idea of dharma also came to be applied to how one fulfills their various duties and obligations in life. *Kula* dharma refers to all the duties we need to fulfill as a part of a family, *varna-ashrama* dharma to the roles according to one's varna and stage in life, and *sva*-dharma to an individual's dharma based on the above factors. Due to the growing influence of Buddhism and Jainism, *sadharana* dharma, defined as all those actions incumbent upon all beings regardless of caste, was considered to be integral in an individual's life. In addition to these, two frameworks built around the manifestation of dharma emerged, *pravritti* and *nivritti* (which will be explored in the following chapters). The principles of dharma were meant to reduce chaos and establish order in a society that was experiencing great flux and expansion through migrations. Even though there was intermingling and coexistence, there were also conflicts between people and tension between the different roles in an individual's lifetime.

The Dharmashastras, codices on law and conduct, furthered the notion of dharma as being specifically based on one's varna, excluding the *mlecchas* or the people who were not a part of the varnas. The epic text Mahabharata explored the tensions, paradoxes, and conflicts between the dharmas. While there was an emphasis on the concept of "ahimsa *paramo* dharma" (non-harming is the highest dharma), there were also times when *himsa* was justified, such as when the social order (varna) was challenged, when righteousness was disrupted, or for one's own survival. In the Vishada Yoga, the first chapter of the Bhagavad Gita, Arjuna is utterly dejected as he faces this existential quandary. To establish justice in the land, he would have to defeat the opposing Kaurava army and inflict violence on many people whom he also loves and reveres.

The early nineteenth century saw another major shift in the meaning and usage of dharma. It came about as a response to the appropriation of the word by Christian missionaries in Bengal, who used it to proclaim Christianity as the "true dharma." For instance, the 1851 Monier Williams dictionary, named after the evangelical British Indologist who compiled it, provided the first meaning of *religion* as dharma.[6] In response to this colonial appropriation of the concept and the expansion of Islam and Christianity in many regions, social reformers like Ram Mohan Roy (Brahmo Samaj in Bengal) and Dayanand Saraswati (Arya Samaj in Punjab) believed it was essential to rid society of the ills of the Hindu religion, like *sati* (the horrific custom of burning the widow on her husband's pyre), idolatry, and child marriage. Both Brahmo Samaj and Arya Samaj were sects within the larger Hindu ecosystem that differed on a few issues, like the emphasis on the Vedas as a primary text (Arya Samaj) and the integration of other traditions (Brahmo Samaj). However, both sects centered their philosophies around the core tenets of Upanishads such as the eminence of formless, universal consciousness. Both sought to unify and revive a diverse, heterogeneous social and religious landscape.

During this time, the expression *sanatan* dharma, or "eternal dharma," became popular,[7] referring to a benevolent form of Hinduism (without the evils of *sati* and child marriage, for example) reclaimed from colonialism. *Sanatan* dharma is often presented as an alternative term to Hindus. Though the term is regarded as an ancient one and was used in a few texts, it was not used in a religious context. There is no treatise specifically on *sanatana* dharma, either as a "conceptual premise or as religious practice, and its occurrence in precolonial India may at best be characterized as sporadic and diverse."[8]

As a two-word compound, the term first makes its appearance in the Buddhist scripture Mahavagga, where truth is extolled as the eternal law into which "the goal and the doctrine are grounded."[9] In the Mahabharata, the great epic exposition on dharma, *sanatan* dharma is used as a compound word 157 times, in a range of contexts, with meanings such as an upholding of truth, being hospitable, and a king's duty to ensure the welfare of his subjects. The term is used in this epic as a "justification of certain behavior or normative ideas—personal, social or religious—prevalent in society,"[10] not as a singular religious or philosophical practice.

The Brahmo and Arya Samaj reformers denounced the caste system to a certain extent, yet did not consider the possibility to abolish it entirely. The Hindu "reform" movements were avowedly nationalistic and anticolonial, mobilizing the masses against Christian missionaries. The movements impacted the savarnas to some extent in terms of challenging superstitions and practices like *sati*, child marriage, and widow remarriage. However, while there was an acknowledgement of the harm of caste oppression, Arya Samaj adherents considered the Vedas to be unequivocally sacred, and they preached accessibility to the teachings of the scriptures. They rejected idol worship and had their own temples and ceremonial practices with priests. There were pathways for folks who were converted to other religions to convert back, but this required a *shuddhikaran* ritual—a purification ceremony with a priest in front of a fire. While some, especially in the northern regions, became Arya Samajis, the underlying implication that one was polluted because of proximity or participation in other religions was rejected by many.

In short, the reform movements were an attempt "to 'dissolve' and not 'annihilate' entrenched caste hierarchy, a definitional subterfuge which would not alter the 'structures of graded inequality at the grassroots.'"[11]

The Genesis of Hinduism as an -ism

In keeping with our root inquiry of the intersection of yoga history and the Hindu religion, there needs to be more clarity about the genesis of the label of "Hindu." This cannot be delved into without contextualizing the "other," i.e., Islam, which was one of the catalysts for the creation of the umbrella term Hindu. India was a region of dynasties, princely states, and republics, in which caste and sectarian allegiance were paramount in one's identity. Faith and spiritual tradition were integral markers, but they were not the only ones. For instance among the important identities were the Vaishnavite (Vishnu worshippers), the Shaivite (Shiva worshippers), the Shakta, the Buddhist, and the Jain. Language and regional affiliations were also important. Ancient India had a profusion of traditions, sects, belief systems, social norms, and, of course, castes. Many of these elements in different permutations and combinations factored into the construction of an individual's identity. There was also fluidity and adaptability between different faith traditions.

Through more than 3,500 years of ancient Indian cultural history, there are vibrant examples of this suppleness that shaped traditions through both integrations and breakaways to create different sects. Within the sramanas, Buddhism had two main schools: the Mahayana (Greater Vehicle) and the Hinayana (Lesser Vehicle). The Jains had their own two main schools, Digambara and Shvetambara, which in turn had many sects. The Vaishnava and the Shaivite had their diversifications, and so did the Shaktas. Each of them had their own followers, their own sects, and in some instances their own formalized religion. This was all in addition to the avarnas, who worshiped their own tree-dwelling *yakshi*s and *grama devata*s, the fierce and benevolent village deities.

So the question arises: When did the label *Hindu* get attached to this legion of peoples? Most importantly, when did the collective see themselves as being a part of a single cohesive conceptual or religious category? While the word *Hindu* may have been used as a contrast to the Islamic presence, the word *Hinduism* became common only in the second quarter of the nineteenth century, mostly due to the British colonial restructuring of Indian society; thus, the word made an appearance in books by British authors.[12] Hindu self-identity expanded from being a solely geographical identification as a general designation for all the people who lived on the banks of the river Sindhu regardless of other affiliations. Its definition expanded to include other sociocultural-religious factors when there was contact with other religious traditions. This contrast especially emerged as a result of "the often antagonistic Hindu and Muslim identities, both individual and communitarian, [that] arose out of political and religious conflicts during the historical periods of the Delhi Sultanate, the Mughal Empire, and the regional Sultanates."[13] Even then there was no reference to Hindu-dharma or Hindu in the ancient Sanskrit texts. While there are not many Sanskrit texts that directly refer to Islam or Muslims other than referring to all who are outside the varnas as *mleccha* or *yavana*, there is more detail about the consciousness of the "other" in north Indian Bhakti poetry.

A fifteenth-century poem by Muslim poet Kabir describes this emergence of a convergence of all the diverse sects, as a contrast against the "other" (referred to below as a Turk, another often-used name for Muslim):

Who is a Hindu, who a Turk?
Both must share a single world.
Koran or Vedas, both read their books.
One has Siva, one Mohammad.
One is a pandit, one a mullah.
Each of them bears a separate name.
But every pot is made from clay.[14]

Kabir eloquently suggests that all are manifestations of the One ("every pot is made from clay") and that the destination is the same (God) even though the paths may vary. In the poem above, one may draw two inferences: The Hindu is perceived as being distinct from Muslim ("one has Shiva, one Mohammed"), and all the many religious traditions other than Islam are grouped together as Hindu. Many of the Bhakti poets used this technique to highlight dogmatism in religion as an obstacle to spiritual emancipation. This also contributed to the growing consciousness of the emerging identity of Hindu.

Even though Hinduism and Islam were distinct, there was also fluidity and intentional exchanges between the traditions, from art and architecture to food and clothing to yoga and some of the tenets within Islam. By the eleventh century, Islam was very integrated into the fabric of the existing Indian tapestry and played a role in the evolution of yoga; thus, it is important for us to know about this connection.

Islam was introduced to the Indian subcontinent in the seventh century through Arab traders on the Malabar and Konkan coasts of India; thus, it was commerce that initially brought Islam to the region. Despite the Arab conquest of Sindh in the latter half of the seventh century CE, the "establishment of Muslim rule in India was a complex and protracted process."[15]

The historian Manu Pillai shares that the oldest Islamic site in Kerala is the Cheraman Jumma Masjid mosque, dated around 629 CE, built during the lifetime of the Prophet Muhammad. The story goes that the mythical ruler of Kerala, Cheraman Perumal, had a dream of the moon splitting into two. The Arab traders who heard of this dream told Perumal that it augured his auspicious pilgrimage to the holy city of Mecca. Heeding their advice, Perumal divided his kingdom among his family and loyal subjects so he could set forth on his pilgrimage. Legend has it that he died as a devout Muslim during his travels, and his friend built the mosque in his name. A text called the Keralolpathi, scribed by a Brahmin, describes this ruler and his embrace of Islam.[16] Thus, the earliest mosque in India bears the name of a Hindu king.

From textual and practice perspectives, there are multiple overlaps among the teachings of Islam, Sufi mystics, and yoga. The rulers of the Delhi Sultanate of northern India (1206–1526) were patrons of Sanskrit intellectuals. During the Mughal dynastic period (from the early sixteenth to the eighteenth centuries), there were many generative interactions as well as violent conflicts between Hindus and Muslims. The Mughals were a Persianate dynasty, meaning that they sponsored Persian as a major language of culture and administration. At the same time, they engaged with Sanskrit scholarship in many ways, they hosted an array of Jain and Brahmin intellectuals at court, and they bestowed titles on members of both communities. This cross-cultural patronage was an integral part of "the public persona of individual kings and members of the Mughal ruling class."[17]

In the 1580s, Emperor Akbar sponsored a translation of the Mahabharata, titled Razmnamah (Book of War), which was integrated into the education of princes. The cross-fertilization of cultures made its way out of royal households into the oral retellings of the epics, infusing them with Islamic flavor. In the Mapilla Ramayana of the Malabar Muslim community of Kerala, references are made to Allah and the shariat, and Ram and Ravana are referred to as Lama and Lavana.[18] During the peak of the Bhakti movement, in the fifteenth century, one comes across a coalescence of faiths among the Sufi *pirs* (people who act as spiritual guides), such as Malik Muhammad Jayasi, who composed devotional poetry in praise of Krishna.

The sixteenth-century Sufi text *Bahr-al-Hayat* describes postures and breathing and meditation techniques, and it has creation myths that are both Quranic and Puranic.[19] In the context of yoga, the Upanishads were translated by Muslim scholars under the patronage of seventeenth-century Mughal king Dara Shikoh, who was deeply interested in the confluence of Vedantic and Sufi thought. On the other hand, his iconoclastic and contro- versial brother Aurangzeb issued repressive edicts like the reimposition of *jaziya* (a military tax for non-Muslims) and other restrictions that aimed to make Islam the dominant religion in his reign. He is believed to have ordered the destruction of a Nath yoga shrine in Gorakhpur and to have built a mosque in its place. Ruthless and ambitious, he ordered the persecution of his brother Dara Shikoh and imprisoned his father, Shah Jahan. He was also interested in the medicine and elixirs developed by the yogis; there are letters between him and the head of the Jakhbar Nath monastery that exhibit an understanding of the monastery's Shaivite lineage.[20] Thus, the relationships between Islamic rulers, yoga, and other spiritual traditions were complex; they were not entirely antagonistic, nor entirely free of strife and violence.

Multiple things can be true at once. It is historically accurate to state that there have been Islamic rulers who were cruel or destroyed monas- teries and temples. It is also true that throughout history there have been other shades and textures of interactions and encounters between Hindus and Muslims, including cultural integration, fierce battles, invasions, and both forced and voluntary conversions to Islam. Caste- and class-oppressed people converted to Islam, Sikhism, and Buddhism because these religions offered pathways for social mobility. However, caste was and is prevalent across all religions of the South Asian countries. Wars have been fought between all religions. These divisions and fissures have not been entirely driven by faith; they have also stemmed from the ambition to expand king- doms and from human greed for power. Art and architecture, literature and poetry are evidence that there always has been a cultural and spiritual synergy among the ancient faiths of the Indian subcontinent, along with wars and conflict. Both are true.

Hinduism was not regarded as a monolithic religion until British colonialists categorized the people they encountered who were not Muslims, who were not Jews, who were not Zorastrians, who were not Christians, as Hindus. The concept of religion itself was a Western one. Integral to this understanding was the necessity of a central canon or set of doctrines as well as allegiance to only one religion at a time. The West—in this case, the British colonizers—framed all other traditions but their own as "religious" or spiritual while treating itself as the default universal or secular tradition. The existing sociospiritual anarchies in colonized India posed grave administrative challenges for the British, who wanted to build strategic political and economic alliances with the ruling elite.

The polarities between Hindus and Muslims were sharpened due to the colonial strategy of homogenizing, essentializing, and universalizing a complex and pluralistic society.[21] The colonialists carried this out by building tactical alliances with the reigning monarchs, categorizing Indigenous cultures, and assiduously constructing the "other." Edward Said's path-breaking book, *Orientalism*, deconstructs the European colonial project of considering the "Orient" (the colonized regions of Asia and Africa) as an object of study, "with an irresistible impulse always to codify, to subdue the infinite variety of the Orient to a complete digest of laws, figures, and customs."[22]

In 1817, James Mill published *The History of British India* despite never having set foot in India and not knowing any of the languages. In accordance with his selective, limited understanding of the dominant dynasties that ruled some of the regions, Mill divided India's history into three major historical periods: ancient Hindu, medieval Muslim, and the colonial period.[23] The book was highly influential during its time and greatly shaped many policies of governance. After its publication, he was offered a position in the East India Company. This work also led to a gross oversimplification of the existing tapestry of religions, castes, sects, and traditions, and the fallacy that the original (ancient) inhabitants of India were a homogeneous entity called the "Hindus" until (medieval) Islamic invasions and European colonialism. The sharp duality of Hindu and Muslim as solidified by the British was the basis for the partition of colonized India into two nations, India and Pakistan, after independence from the British in 1947.

During the eighteenth century, European scholars evinced curiosity about the history of India, and they turned to their sources of information—the Brahmin priests whom they regarded as the "guardians of the ancient tradition," which were "preserved in the Sanskrit sources with which only they were familiar."[24] The British selectively sponsored translations of Sanskrit texts such as the Vedas, the Upanishads, and the Bhagavad Gita, as they were thought to be representative of the intellectual elite. Max Mueller—an influential nineteenth-century German-born naturalized citizen of Britain, who was a professor of comparative philology and religious studies at Oxford—projected the value of a monotheistic religion based on his own Protestant upbringing. He studied Sanskrit and the Vedas, and he translated the Upanishads. He advanced a thesis that the Vedas represented somewhat of a peak of intellect; but still, the people were in need of colonial intervention.[25] He asserted that the Vedic period was the Hindu golden age, and he urged Hindus to return to the Vedas to reclaim the purity of their tradition. There was an emphasis on a common ancestry with the Indo-Aryans, and Vedic worship of nature-based deities was linked to European romanticism. His work amplified the Vedic teachings as the root of Indian religion.

The colonially sanctioned Eurocentric notions of a monolithic religion went a long way toward diminishing the heterogeneity of narratives and the lived experiences of different castes, sects, and faith traditions. The reconfiguration of "Hinduism" as a monolithic religion amplified the laws, traditions, and principles of only one section of society, the savarnas, even though they were not the majority. The avarnas practiced their own religions and followed their own spiritual practices that were oral and often not recorded in writing and/or in Sanskrit. Many of these constructions of a homogenous

Hindu identity were uplifted by philosophers like Vivekananda and other anticolonial nationalists, who were eager to unite a fractured, disenfranchised people against the might of the British empire.

The foreign concept of religion was institutionalized in India during the colonial period through the "agency of the British census."[26] The first such nationwide census took place in 1881, and its categories were arbitrary based on a Western understanding of religion rather than a reflection of the ground realities of colonized India. For instance, in Punjab, Sikhs were included as Hindus until 1868, and when that identification was ignored, a new category of Sikh-Hindu was introduced. Today they are considered two completely different religions. Many traditions that had amorphous origins later coalesced for various reasons, including colonial restructurings, and they continued to solidify.

Religions are not created in isolation; nor do they gather momentum without institutional support. Many religions therefore faded as they attracted fewer adherents. Buddhism in India, for instance, started out as a highly popular religion, as it was more egalitarian than Brahmanism; but today it is practiced by only 0.7 percent of the population.[27] The reasons are many: Buddhism was mostly monastic and became more esoteric with scholars sequestered in monasteries, who were thus less connected to public life than other religions of the time. There was a gradual tapering off of royal patronage and thus a loss of institutional support.

Contemporary mainstream yoga studies exclude the interwoven histories of religions, colonialism, and castes. Yoga is situated within and without the texts and tenets of different religions, with caste as the common denominator. Scholars differ on the centrality of yoga in various religions, especially Hinduism, Buddhism, and Jainism. Some argue that it forms the very essence of those religions, while others downplay its importance and merely nod at its presence within those religions. Erasure, denial, or ignorance of the complexity ensures that dominant narratives of yoga as solely physical and/or yoga as a Hindu practice get amplified. As discerning yoga practitioners, we can continually seek out and learn from the myriad intersections of our ancestral discoveries, learnings, and explorations into healing and liberation, while being rooted in our own paths.

What Even Is Yoga?

What even is yoga? I often begin teaching with this question because there is no single definition; rather, there are many, and they are often contradictory. Most popular wellness magazines would define yoga as a union of mind, body, and spirit, but this is misleading and simplistic. Yoga is an umbrella term used for different schools of thought, consisting of a multilayered and often contradictory collection of practices encompassing various branches, cultures, and traditions. Before we get into the history, it is important to know a few key definitions of yoga as they are mentioned in some of the central texts. This in itself is challenging because the underlying themes of the teachings are varied and multidimensional, and the sources are expansive, coming from a breadth of philosophers, sages, thinkers, and scholars.

The term *yoga* is a multivalent word used to refer to many things: practices, disciplines, states of being, ways of living, and paths toward transcendence. Thus, a polythetic approach, which recognizes similar features in concepts and a family of resemblances,[28] is a useful tool for defining yoga. The root word of yoga is *yuj*, meaning to yoke or to join. This imagery of the yoke comes from Vedic literature and refers to the horse and the chariot or oxen yoked to a cart or plow. The metaphor becomes very familiar, as it is mentioned often in the Upanishads and the Bhagavad Gita, where it is used as a symbolic representation of the connection between the mind, the senses, and consciousness. Even though the word *yoga* does not make an appearance until a few centuries later, there are textual references to yoga in the oldest Sanskrit composition, the Rig Veda (composed between 1500–1200 BCE), that indicate the use of visionary meditation. This work also includes a hymn suggesting a mystical ascetic tradition.[29]

Around 500 BCE, sramanas (strivers) and *vratyas* (wandering ascetics who lived on the borders of Vedic society) challenged and rejected the rigid ritualism of the emerging power constructs propagated by Vedic Brahmanism. The goal of sramanic striving was the attainment of moksha (liberation) from the cycles of birth and death (samsara). This was in stark contrast to the ascetics of the Vedic tradition, who also practiced *tapas* (austerity) to obtain more material and worldly goals, like power (*bala*), supernatural abilities, or victory over a rival kingdom. Buddha's life story includes his experiences practicing with such ascetics. The fourth century BCE travel accounts of Alexander the Great shed light on some of these mendicants who stood on one leg, enduring great heat and cold alike. Therefore, we know that spiritual aspirations included psychophysical practices even before the word *yoga* was mentioned in formal texts. While sramanas were independent of the Vedic traditions, they also influenced Vedic development. Thus, there were Vedic sages as well as sramanic renunciates, and both evolved techniques of dhyana (meditation), concepts and traditions that later came to be known as yoga.

The roots of yoga were thus complex, with both heterodox and orthodox elements. While the teachings of the Vedas and the Upanishads were integral streams in the ocean of yoga, heterodox sramanas challenged the sacrificial rituals and hierarchies of Vedic people. Gautam Buddha and Vardhamana Mahavira (the great Jain *thirthankara*, or guru) were both savarnas, yet they rejected caste-oriented hierarchies. The sramanas renounced material possessions and were dependent for food and sometimes shelter on the people of the region. They accepted food from all castes without exception. While some were solitary seekers of salvation in forests and caves, others were more engaged in sociopolitical activities, building places of gathering and education like monasteries, stupas, and viharas. They were deeply concerned with teaching ethical codes of conduct, vociferously criticized those who flouted the rules, and challenged the existing sociopolitical institutions.

One of the earliest mentions of yoga is in the Katha Upanishad, in which yoga is described as a means of meditation through which the seeker can comprehend Atma as Brahman. The teachings emerge through a conversation between a precocious boy, Nachiketa, and Yama, the god of death. Esoteric and existential themes are explored, and concepts of consciousness, immortality, and the meaning of life are revealed through lyrical allegories that are typical of the Upanishads. Such stylistic and conceptual components are repeated often and developed further in other texts, such as the Gita and the Yoga Sutras. For instance, the body is compared to the chariot, the *buddhi* (intellect) is the charioteer, the passenger in the chariot is the individual self or Atma, the senses (*indriya*s) are the horses, and the reins are the mind (*manas*). The Katha Upanishad offers one of the first clear definitions of yoga as a practice with a goal, in which the focus is on cultivation of restraint of the senses and thereby liberation from cycles of rebirth: "When the five senses [*jnanani*], along with the mind, remain still and the intellect is not active, that is known as the highest state. They consider yoga to be a firm restraint of the senses" (Katha Upanishad 6.10).[30]

Patanjali's Yoga Sutra teaches yoga practitioners to seek freedom from an overidentification with and attachment to prakriti, or manifest nature. This definition of yoga is very close to the Pali Buddhist texts (500–100 CE), in which yoga is referred to as a discipline, a form of asceticism that offers methods for achieving prime concentration of the senses. The ultimate goal is the eventual liberation (nirvana) from our attachment to the phenomenal world. In Jain philosophy (500–300 BCE), the teachings refer to *gunasthana*, stages of virtue, and to yoga as a practice of progressing through the stages to gain samadhi.

The Yoga Sutras of Patanjali (composed around 100 CE) define yoga as the cessation of the fluctuations of the mind (*citta vritti nirodhah*). The text's often terse aphorisms offer a practical pathway into the theory of the dualistic Samkhya system, which has two main categorically distinct principles: purusa as the omniscient, omnipresent, unmanifest consciousness, and prakriti as manifest, ever-changing nature. Patanjali systematically codifies the practices into ashtanga (meaning the eight *anga*s or limbs of yoga), where the practitioner is instructed to traverse from the *bahiranga* (outer realms) to the *antaranga* (inner realms) so as to gain *kaivalya*, liberation or isolation of prakriti from purusa. *Yama*s and *niyama*s, the ethical and moral codes, are the first two *anga*s. They are the commencement in the yogic journey that both acknowledges and foregrounds social-emotional-psychological goals with spiritual aspiration. Thus, the aspirant's responsibilities are directed toward the cocreation of a just and compassionate world, an optimal environment to pursue the personal goal of liberation. One of the central teachings of the Yoga Sutras is about *avidya* (ignorance) of our essence, our *purusha vishesha*, or the Special Self. Patanjali's explanation of *kriya* yoga directs the *abhyasa* (practice) to gain liberation from an identification with the mind and body through discipline (*tapas*), self-study (*svadhyaya*), and surrender to Ishvara (Sutra 2.1).

A parallel pathway to austere asceticism was offered by what is known as Tantra, a world-affirming philosophy that originated around 500 CE. *Tantra* comes from the word *tan*, which means to weave together a complex web of rituals and practices propounding Tantrashastras. Tantras are believed to have originated from ascetic groups living on the margins of society, in cremation grounds or *shmashana*. Tantra subverted Vedic orthodoxy as well as sramanic renunciation with a fervent reverence for all material aspects of the world, including the taboo and macabre, as manifestations of the divine. Women, Shudras, and avarnas were active participants, agents of enlightenment as well as sources of enormous power. Women were teachers and partners in sexual rites, and seminal fluids were considered the distillation of Shakti; however, the texts were written from a male perspective.[31]

Tantric practices connected esoteric realms with every aspect of the human experience and honed in on both subtle anatomy and the gross body as microcosms of all of creation. The body was conceived as composed of prana (vital life energy) that flows through channels (*nadis*) and centers (chakras), with a mystical envisioning of powerful kundalini energy as a coiled serpent at the base of the spine. There is no single monolithic form of tantra as the practices were developed along with and interspersed throughout Buddhist, Jain, Saiva, Vaishnava, and Shakta traditions; thus, they overlapped with both the atheistic and theistic systems.

In the Bhagavad Gita, the term *yoga* appears 150 times, both as praxis and as states of being. Krishna shares that yoga is both a state of being (*samatvam* or equanimity) and ways of doing (*karmasu kausalam*, or skill in action). Yoga is also a path or *marga* (karma, *jnana*, or bhakti) toward liberation, moksha. Yoga is the way to Atma-*jnana* (knowledge of our true nature). There is an integration of the teachings of Samkhya with Upanishadic insight. The Bhagavad Gita was composed at a time when Brahmanic householder religion was challenged by Buddhist, Jain, and sramanic traditions. In order to appeal to the householder while emphasizing societal order or one's role in society as determined by one's varna, the tenets of dharma and karma were delved into with great detail. Krishna reiterates the agency and the sovereignty of the seeker, who is presented with different but equal paths that in turn render an ease and accessibility to transcendental ambition. Bhakti *marga* (or yoga), the path of loving devotion, is one of the primary ways in which religions interact with yoga.

Both Upanishadic and Patanjala yoga give a minimal nod to asana. There are a couple of passages in the Yoga Sutras that refer to it as a posture/seat for meditation and the need for ease and stability. This does not mean, however, that the austerities did not include physical practice; the Mahabharata and even Buddhist lore describe several physical practices, such as meditating while standing on one foot or raising a hand for years. However, there is no text in the first ten centuries of the millennium that systematically elaborates on the physical practices until the composition of texts from hatha yoga traditions that expound upon the practices of physical yoga.

Hatha, meaning force, refers to the physical austerities practiced by yogis who are not necessarily renunciates. This tradition begins to be developed more formally by the end of the first millennium CE.[32] In the hatha yoga tradition, the body becomes a transmutative tool, something to gain mastery of so as to obtain powers, both mystical and manifest. The practices of hatha yoga include cleansing techniques (*satkarmas*), asanas, and methods for harnessing prana through breath (pranayama) and body (mudra). Health, longevity, and immortality are sought through these practices. While many hatha yoga practices are referred to in several textual sources, such as the eleventh-century Tantric text *Amritasiddhi*, it is the thirteenth-century

Vaishnavite text *Dattatreyayogasastra* that first systematizes hatha yoga, and the fifteenth-century *Hatha Yoga Pradipika* and *Gherandasamhita* that expand and elaborate the field of physical practices.

Hatha yoga and Patanjali's yoga converge at various points. The most recent intersection is at the end of the eighteenth century, when yoga goes through a renaissance of sorts through the teachings of Swami Vivekananda, the charismatic monk-saint from Bengal, and Tirumalai Krishnamacharya (often called the father of modern yoga), a Brahmin scholar-yogi whose famous students—B. K. S. Iyengar, Indra Devi, Pattabhi Jois, and Desikachar—innovated and propounded their own yogic lineages. Most contemporary transnational yoga is deeply influenced by these lineages. Chapter 5 will explore the complex power dynamics of the guru relationship in the context of yoga.

All the source texts have been studied through ancient and contemporary commentaries. Most of us in modern yoga are students of translations of those commentaries. For example, Vyasa's commentary on Patanjali's Yoga Sutras are the most influential commentaries that have been translated. The eighth-century scholar Sankaracharya's commentaries on the Upanishads are considered to be the most influential in the explication of Advaita Vedanta. Most of the ancient commentaries of texts were written in Sanskrit by Brahmin men. The more modern ones are in European languages, again written by men. This is an important and unnamed lens through which we yoga practitioners receive the teachings today. If there were compositions or yogic practices by and for women, avarnas, and gender minorities, they either have not yet been discovered or have been absorbed into the larger textual corpus.

Yoga Is a Many-Splendored Thing

To come to a shared understanding of what yoga is, we have to explore some of the central inquiries that our ancestors dwelled on for centuries. Yoga is a many-splendored thing because approaches to central queries differ greatly between traditions. For instance, questions about the relationship between consciousness and matter vary greatly in the ancient commentaries on the Upanishads. The Vedantic approach gleaned from the Upanishads regards pure individual consciousness (*jivatma*) as a reflection of Brahman or Param-atma (universal consciousness). Thus, per the Upanishads, yoga is referred to as union of individual spirit/consciousness or Atma with the perennial spirit/consciousness, Param-atma. On the other hand, the dualistic Samkhya-informed Yoga Sutras define yoga as the practices that lead to isolation or disjunction of purusa and prakriti. The hatha and tantra yoga traditions center the body as a vehicle for alchemical transformation of gross and subtle energies. As we can see from the various histories and intersections in this chapter, yoga is not a single idea but a concurrence of many teachings. Following are a few broad commonalities and themes that course through these teachings, even though they may differ on the how and the why:

- We are all deeply, viscerally, and spiritually interconnected sentient beings infused with consciousness.

- The practice of yoga cultivates discernment about our mind-body identification and *samskaras* of attachment.

- *Dukka* or human suffering is inevitable.

- The solutions for liberation from suffering, though varied, are available to those who seek with dedication through *sadhana*.

- The physical-emotional-intellectual body or embodiment can be a source of salvation (in bhakti, hatha, and tantra traditions).

Liberation—also referred as *mukti*, *kaivalya*, or moksha—is thus the aim of yoga. The paths to this elusive, aspirational, and emancipated state may vary, but the teachings acknowledge a deep yearning within to expand our awareness of how we can free ourselves from our identification with the ever-changing material realm. The practices delve into how we can find release from physical-emotional-mental and spiritual suffering, to know and be in our truest essence. Yoga is a revelation of our primordial nature, which is beyond the limitations of individual mind-ego and sociocultural conditioning.

Although most of us in the contemporary world may not have the focus of gaining salvation as people did in bygone times (who can pursue moksha while navigating capitalism?), most of us are seeking to reduce and transcend *dukka*, our suffering, in some way. We long to be happy, to be healthy, to gain clarity of purpose and meaning in our everyday lives. We long to belong. Faith anchors us in the wild currents of a world that is increasingly challenging, violent, and complex. Most of us are engaged in the world, filled with the messiness of relationships and transactions. There is a yearning to find our ways out of intertwined oppressive systems that are desecrating the earth and dehumanizing each other in every way. Many of us are seeking a radical reimagination of the world we live in.

We will delve into an exploration of this quest for individual and collective transformation. Each chapter will use a story from a specific period about folks who challenged dominant culture and voiced radical dissent within the yogic traditions—bright sparks from the past who continue to light up our paths today. Each of their quests stems from a different spiritual and philosophical approach, a different way of seeking the divine. While Sulabha is a *jnani* ascetic, Radha, Akka Mahadevi, and Piro portray the vastness, complexity, and diversity of the bhakti *marga*. Thus, when the word *yoga* is used in the next four stories, it refers to the bhakti and *jnana* aspects of the larger Yoga tradition. I hope they ignite personal inquiry and offer nourishing insight into what lies within and around us.

Key Takeaways

Embrace the Luminous Threads of Pluralism

The Muslim and the Hindu today are often pitted against one another, emphasizing the violence of historical imperialism. There is rampant erasure or rewriting of history to suit ethnonationalist agendas in India and the diaspora, and that translates into yoga spaces. In India's 2023–24 high school history syllabus, vast portions of the Mughal legacy have been completely erased.[33] This is a part of the strategy to portray India as a historically homogenous Hindu nation. Not only is this grossly misleading, it erases the countless ways in which the two religious and cultural traditions have also coexisted. Yes, there has been violence and conflict between the two; there also has been a blending and merging, and this aspect needs to be reclaimed in all ways possible.

There are many historical examples of the synergies between Islam and yoga, including some from the Mughal period that pertain to yoga texts and bhakti practices like pilgrimage to holy sites. For instance, there are many paintings during this period that depict yogis. Some are Nath yogis with their typical earrings that loop through the lower part of the ear to surround the entire earlobe, and others are shown with *yogapatta*s, or "straps." There is also one from the 1500s that shows ascetics being shaved. During Shah Jahan's rule in the sixteenth century, Kavindracharya Sarasvati successfully convinced the Mughal king to rescind a tax on Hindu pilgrims to Benares and Prayag.[34] The Mahabharata, an epic from a Vaishnavite tradition, was taught to sixteenth-century Mughal princes as lessons in the craft of warfare.

Referring back to the metaphor of the *godhadi* (quilt or tapestry), the threads of the past surface in different incarnations. Ideas and concepts also shift and adapt to changes in society. The principle of dharma that referred to ritualistic actions in the Vedic period changed to mean "righteousness," and then the definition of righteousness itself was based on one's social position in the caste and gender hierarchy. By studying the history of a concept or a text, we know more about the values of our ancestors—what they considered important or precious, or conversely, disposable and unimportant—and by knowing them more, we know ourselves. The tapestry of yoga history can be a catalyst in embodying an inherent interconnectedness, especially now when yoga is operationalized to support ethnonationalist agendas.

Pluralism does not mean we are all the same, or even that we agree all the time. It means we are cognizant of our differences, and we acknowledge the unique contributions and perspectives of diverse lived experiences. This does not exclude conflict; there are tensions and contradictions, paradoxes that can reveal deeper levels of understanding of our own biases. Dissent and disagreement, debate and counterarguments are a part of our spiritual-intellectual DNA—a fact that is glossed over by dominant cultural institutions that encourage and reward conformity. We need to unravel our deeply embedded *samskaras*, which may be daunting; yet this is critical if we are to disrupt the past and ongoing *himsa* of caste and religious hegemony.

Every act of understanding furthers our own self-knowledge. Each glimpse of a new possibility is also an understanding of our own possibilities.[35] This aspect of self-awareness elucidates the potential we have, as sentient beings, to embrace complexity within both ourselves and the other. In a world that is increasingly polarized in every way, we can lean into the fluidity of cultures as windows of insight into heterogeneity and acceptance. This approach can be an antidote to the imposed pseudouniformity of increasingly homogenized cultures. Nothing is created in isolation; the concept of purity—of a people, a practice, a concept—is a fallacy. In truth, practices, concepts, systems, religions, and institutions are built from their predecessors. This notion of collective creation can shift power constructs regarding who is considered as an owner and an expert, and why.

Syncretism—defined as the "the attempt to combine opposing doctrines and practices, especially in reference to philosophical and religious systems"[36]—and hybridity are more common than dominant cultures will admit. In an increasingly fractured world, where social media algorithms entrench us in silos, leaning into the varied contributions that form the foundations of healing practices can heal communal wounds and disrupt hegemony. We will explore syncretism in greater detail in chapters 5 and 6. The dominance of the Hindu Brahminical narratives in yoga is a reflection of the broader historical and current political contexts of the region. However, that does not mean yoga is only Hindu. Yoga predates organized religions and was birthed by radical ascetics who rejected rituals and hierarchies. It goes back to a time before the word *Hindu* was coined. Its teachings have been infused with different religions and worldviews and have in turn influenced cultures. The weaving together of this multihued, multithread tapestry has the potential to offer much solace and inspiration for the world as it sheds light on the struggles, foibles, and triumphs of our ancestors.

Indigeneity Is Complex

Hinduism is a porous system rather than an intractable religion, and it referred to many cultural groups in a geographic location. The texts such as the Vedas that many identify as significant to their spiritual lineages were not "Indigenous" to the land, as Indigeneity itself is complicated. The notion that India was originally Hindu until Muslim invaders came into the "country" is erroneously simplistic. There was a plethora of belief systems, deities, and traditions that coalesced to form what is now known as the Hindu religion. The word *Hindu* was a designation of geographical identity and was not used as a cultural or religious marker until Islamic imperialism and British colonialism. India is a land of many migrations, intermingling, integration, invasions, and conflicts between those who arrived in the land as nomads, traders, invaders, or colonizers. Most of its people are thus of mixed ancestry. The societal undergirding for the Indic region is the caste system that pervades all major religions, like Hinduism, Islam, Christianity, and Sikhism.

Appropriation and Appreciation of Yoga Are Not Binary Constructs

Cultural (mis-) appropriation occurs in the context of a power dynamic, so it is not entirely an innocent action of assimilation or adoption. Rather, it refers to the "taking of intellectual property, traditional knowledge, cultural expressions, or artifacts from someone else's culture without permission. This can include unauthorized use of another culture's dance, dress, music, language, folklore, cuisine, traditional medicine, religious symbols, etc. It's most likely to be harmful when the source community is a minority group that has been oppressed or exploited in other ways or when the object of appropriation is particularly sensitive, e.g. sacred objects."[37] The gap in power and privilege is an important factor that is often understated when presenting appreciation as a supposed antidote for appropriation. Appreciation does not entirely heal the wounds of historical oppression. We need more intentional conduits for trust, building relationships and solidarities across differences.

Dominant culture thrives on binaries; thus, complexity and nuance are missed entirely in discussions of appropriation of yoga in the West. In the context of yoga, the opposite of appropriation is not only appreciation; it is also unraveling the threads of power and hegemony that run through the tapestry of yoga. While there are many folks, especially from the South Asian diaspora, taking a stance against the commodification and appropriation of yoga by the West, the discussions have been limited to a West vs. East binary. However, this simplistic rhetoric does not account for the dynamism of the globalization of culture. While it's important to disrupt dominant neoliberal narratives in yoga, there is much denial and ignorance of a compelling need to acknowledge the dominance of Brahmanism and the impact of religious extremism in yoga traditions and lineages.

By glossing over the heterogeneity in South Asian cultures and the heterodoxy in religious and spiritual traditions, yoga practitioners lose out on the richness of multiple wisdom streams. By not acknowledging historical and ongoing Brahmanical hegemony, as savarnas we deny or ignore the lived experiences of people impacted by caste oppression.

As anticaste activist and writer Prachi Patankar asserts:

> It should not be assumed that all the Dalit, Bahujan, Adivasi, Muslim, Christian, Buddhist, or Sikh communities embrace brahmanical forms of yoga as part of their culture. Representing South Asia as the birthplace of a mythical homogeneous culture is a crusade of the chauvinistic upper-caste Hindus. We need to consciously learn about and highlight the rich, diverse cultures, histories, customs, and spiritual practices of the vast majority of people in South Asia, especially the Dalit and Adivasi communities who are continuing to struggle to keep their cultures alive. What we need is a constant challenge to the caste-privileged attempt to define Hindu, Indian, or South Asian culture as monoliths.[38]

We need to not only study the teachings of yoga in context of the time of their development; we also need to dig through how these teachings have been used to maintain systems of oppression throughout history. Sifting through the teachings with a critical lens and discerning the historical constructs of power is imperative if we are to heal the wounds of separation. Yoga has the potential to reduce physical, psychological, and spiritual suffering (*dukka*) and build community, but yoga spaces are a microcosm of dominant cultures everywhere and have been operationalized to maintain power constructs of caste, religion, race, class, and ability. Therefore, mere appreciation of a culture is not enough; we have to go one step further and discard the elements that have caused oppression, like caste and patriarchy. Just as we discern the impact of our communication on the other, not merely our intention, we, as yoga practitioners in the complex modern world, have to cultivate the same introspection regarding the impact of texts, doctrines, and practices that have harmed and continue to harm millions.

Depending on our positionality, skill, and lived experiences, each of us has a role to play in challenging white supremacy and caste supremacy. Both of these phenomena operate in modern yoga, albeit in different ways. As a non–South Asian yoga practitioner, one can cultivate authentic relationships with folks from the source cultures, in addition to studying and centering voices that are erased in Western yoga. Representation matters for people who have been historically erased and marginalized. Seeing oneself in a position of power and expertise is in itself powerful and healing.

If you are a white yoga practitioner, how can you be an advocate for diverse voices and perspectives in your yoga spaces, as teachers, experts, mentors, or authors? How can you challenge deeply held biases about the "other"? Yoga as a fitness and wellness modality is an outcome of colonization and capitalism. How can you leverage your proximity to power and privilege to intentionally shift this notion? How can self and the collective be visualized as a sacred continuum, not as separate entities? How can we hold the tension inherent in the fact that our lived experiences matter and shape our inner lives and outer worlds?

As a savarna yoga practitioner, it is my responsibility to study caste histories in all their mediums—written, narrated, or sung by the folks from those communities—because many of these stories have been erased by educational institutions shaped by the dominant culture. Building authentic relationships of trust across differences takes time, effort, and consistency. True accountability involves not only apologizing but also understanding the impact your actions have had on yourself and others. It also includes reparations to the harmed parties; but most importantly, "true accountability is changing your behavior so that the harm, violence, abuse does not happen."[39] Writer and activist Mia Mingus has developed a four-part model of accountability, working from a framework of transformative justice. I offer these four queries from her work to support ongoing points of inquiry:

- **Self-reflection:** How is our attachment to comfort holding us back from the practice of radical truth telling (*satya*)? How can we speak up about the prevalence of caste, race, class, gender, and ability supremacy in our yoga spaces?

- **Apology:** How can we acknowledge past and ongoing harm that we have actively or unknowingly propagated in yoga spaces? How can we apologize in small and big ways?

- **Repair:** How can we make amends/build trust to cocreate a community that supports and nourishes, and does not punish dissenting voices?

- **Changed behavior:** How can we shift resources, share spaces, and center marginalized voices, thus leaning into the yogic teachings of the interconnectedness of all creation?

3

SULABHA,
THE REBELLIOUS
PHILOSOPHER

The secret of the Great Stories is that they have no secrets. The Great Stories are the ones you have heard and want to hear again. The ones you can enter anywhere and inhabit comfortably. They don't deceive you with thrills and trick endings. They don't surprise you with the unforeseen. They are as familiar as the house you live in. Or the smell of your lover's skin. You know how they end, yet you listen as though you don't. In the way that although you know that one day you will die, you live as though you won't. In the Great Stories you know who lives, who dies, who finds love, who doesn't. And yet you want to know again.

—ARUNDATHI ROY, *The God of Small Things*

Rays of light seem to emanate from her eyes, all-seeing, all-knowing, all-being. She walks with her feet barely touching the earth, as if belonging to neither the earth nor the heavens, as if coming from another dimension altogether. She is completely at ease with who she is, unapologetic in her autonomy, her head high, shoulders relaxed, her visage attentive and receptive to all that she hears and sees in a room full of men, learned and powerful. She has taken on this physical form, beguiling in its youth and appearance, for a specific purpose; she can morph into any shape she chooses. She has heard of the mighty King Janaka of Mithila, a householder and ruler who claims to have gained moksha, emancipation from the cycles of birth and death, and she wants to ascertain for herself if this is true indeed. So here she is in person, ready to engage in philosophical debate. She is Sulabha; the scene is King Janaka's court.

King Janaka, the learned one, the powerful one, sees the radiant young woman and welcomes her into his court filled with great sages. He offers her a seat among those respected across the lands for their insight into the sacred texts. They are present for the Great Debate; the knowledge that emerges from such a debate, vadavidya, will inform and teach the rest of the world about life and living, salvation and the Brahman, about thought and experience. Great wisdom will emerge from debates such as these. He is intrigued with her poise, her youth, her assured demeanor. But then he senses something. Sulabha is using her yogic siddhi *(power) to "look" into his consciousness to gauge if he has indeed gained moksha as he claims to have. Janaka is shaken by this deep examination by someone so young, and a woman at that! His ego bruised, his civility dissipates as he reprimands her, asking her who she belongs to and how dare she, a young woman, challenge him, he who is the most revered scholar of them all.*

Sulabha cleverly turns his egotistical bragging into pointing out how one's physical body is subject to the laws of karma and changes every instant, how every being is infused with immutable spirit/Atma and has the potential for liberation, and that he cannot hold her gender or her youth against her. She proceeds with clarity to say that the Self, the Atma, has no gender, it is the physical body that shows one's biological sex, and that gender is fluid and can change during one's lifetime. She calls him out, saying he, as a self-professed wise scholar, a yogi, should have known that. Janaka is startled with the depth of her knowledge, aggrieved that she seems to be getting ahead of him, and falls silent, indicating that she is the winner in the debate.

Sulabha is a *rishika* or woman ascetic, a scholar and a Kshatriya, a symbolic figure, a character who is referred to in many texts. The earliest reference to her is from the Vedic period, in the Saulubha Shakha, which is ascribed to her. She is depicted as a revered teacher in the Kaushitaki Brahmana, although her most important appearance as a character is in the Shanti Parva of the epic Mahabharata, where she enters into a debate with King Janaka.[1] When I first read about her in the work of scholar and activist Ruth Vanita, I was astounded at her incisive and radical thoughts—for then and now! She stands out as a rebellious philosopher in more ways than one. She is a single woman, learned in the texts, a *yogini* (a female spiritual practitioner with mystical powers or siddhis) who could transform herself and roam the earth with freedom. Her knowledge and intellect were above par, cutting across complex issues of philosophy, gender, language, and thought.

In Sanskrit *Sulabha* means accessible or natural, perhaps alluding to her steadfastness of being at ease. She was not a Brahmin by birth; rather, she was a Kshatriya who renounced the material world and marriage in favor of intellectual and spiritual pursuits. She is not as well-known as a few other women scholars who are mentioned in the Upanishads, like Gargi and Maitreyi. Sulabha is victorious in her encounter with Janaka as she expounds with immense clarity of thought and insight upon the true nature of Atma and Brahman, individual and eternal consciousness, the ultimate teachings of the Upanishads. Her sagacity and intellectual prowess in distinguishing between gender and sex is really vital in the world today when gender is grossly misunderstood, institutionalized, and governed in binaries.

Sulabha's tenacity in speaking truth to power, calling out a mighty king in his own court, is a lesson in courage; and yet her contribution and startling brilliance are not referred to by many scholars or others who know the stories of the Mahabharata. Why not? Was it because most women of her time belonged to their fathers, husbands, sons, or brothers, but she says she belonged to no one? She is unique here, as most of the women ascetics begin that path after their husbands become rishis or *sanyasi*s. Was it because she was single during a time when a woman's spiritual success was measured by their devotion to men or gods? Was it because she defeated a powerful king, not with the fierce weapons and physical valor of a goddess, but by her mental prowess, the realm of men then (and now)? Was it because her controversial and disruptive thoughts expressed in the debate were uncomfortable and dangerous to repeat and perpetuate?

Sulabha is described as a *tapasvini* (a woman who practices austerities), a *rishika* (ascetic) who is calm at all times. Even when Janaka confronts her, she answers with poise and clarity, hallmarks of a truly Self-realized person or Atma-*jnani*. Sulabha's debate is located in the Shanti Parva book of the Mahabharata, whose authorship is attributed to Krishna Dvaipayana, also known as Vyasa. Vyasa is of mixed-varna parentage: His father was a Brahmin, and his mother was the daughter of a fisherman. The Mahabharata was compiled at a time when there was both fluidity and conflict between the varnas, in addition to tension between the ascetic and householder traditions. This dialectical struggle between the two traditions is reflected not only in Vyasa's own life but also in the characterizations of Sulabha and Janaka. Sulabha is a renunciate Kshatriya, free from worldly attachments, who is now a yogini. Janaka is a married king and a scholar well-versed in all the texts who claims to have achieved moksha. This demonstrates a fluidity between the varnas, suggesting a person's agency in choosing how they want to live and achieve moksha. The dichotomy of approaches to salvation is important for understanding the placement of caste and gender.

Within this chapter, we will look at some key concepts embedded in the debate that highlight Sulabha's thoughts on the difference between body and Atma. It is important to be careful to not impose our modern understanding of equity, equality, and gender fluidity on a debate that was recorded thousands of years ago. However, the debate emphasizes some of the core teachings of the Upanishads that can help modern yoga practitioners navigate notions about gender that persist even today.

"The Self has no gender."[2] The Self or Atma is the spirit that infuses all of creation and has no gender. Sulabha says that all of creation is prakriti. Primordial nature gets manifested and expressed as *vyakta* (Sanskrit for "expression"). The physical, mental, and emotional dimensions of *vyakta* are ever changing and are not stable entities. The physical body is sexed, and that too changes during our lifetime. In great detail, Sulabha describes the different developmental phases of a fetus in the womb, showing that one's biology is different from one's gender. She delves into the stage at nine months when the reproductive organs become visible and the fetus gets a name and form (*nama-rupa*). Just like everything else, gender is not a constant; it can change and is fluid. She makes the distinction between sex and gender and states that both are in flux and thus subject to change. The Atma, on the other hand is eternal and does not change.

All beings are equal, made up of the same constituents, and can achieve moksha. Since all of creation has the same Atma, anyone regardless of their varna or gender can aspire to moksha. Sulabha explains that all bodies are made up of the same elements, the same particles that are in constant motion and flux and are constantly changing. She calmly states that since the mind and body have no fixed identity, Janaka's questioning is ignorant, as he mistakenly refers to all the attributes of one's physical body (outward appearance) as one's identity.

***Varna-ashramas* are labels, and subject to change.** In response to Janaka's assertion that he is an emancipated, learned king, while she is a beautiful, young woman incapable of such wisdom, she points out that being what she is doesn't mean she cannot be as learned or as wise as he is. She then asserts that a truly "evolved" or self-realized person recognizes the oneness of all things and does not judge anyone based on their physical body, marital status, varna, or gender. When Janaka sees her, he assumes she is a Brahmin ascetic because of her simple garb and ease of countenance, and he angrily accuses her of entering his consciousness without consent, thus causing a mixed-varna union. Sulabha points out that the true self is beyond the categorization of varna, age, and gender, and that he is confused between a spiritual and a sexual engagement. She points out that she was ascertaining if his claim of moksha was indeed true, which does not have anything to do with his physical body.

The Ascetic and the Householder

Sulabha is an ascetic. As a renunciate, her dharma is to pursue the goal of moksha without any attachment to worldly pleasures or personal relationships. If she were a householder, Janaka's questioning of who she belonged to may have been more relevant, as it might have been a reference to her role in the family and the larger community. One of the key frameworks to contextualize this discussion on the dynamics of gender and dharma is pravritti dharma and nivritti dharma.

Pravritti (turning toward) dharma is the way of the householder, in which individuals actively pursue reciprocal relationships with each other. Pravritti dharma contextualizes individuals and as scholar Arti Dhand states, "situates them relationally on the interlocking matrices of gender, age, occupation" and "embraces all aspects of social relationships."[3] In the pravritti mode of life, there is an acknowledgement of interdependence, where everything and everyone has a place so as to maintain harmony in all of creation. This tradition necessitates a preservation and perpetuation of order and thus the emphasis and regard of varna (class) and ashrama (stage in a person's life) dharma. Each human therefore enacts their responsibility in the collective and performs their duties with dedication to receive salvation through karma (action).

In the pravritti mode, the pursuit of dharma (right conduct as per one's varna and ashrama), *artha* (livelihood), *kama* (pleasure) and moksha (liberation) are emphasized as the four *purushartha*s or life goals. Thus, there is a place given to worldly pursuits such as gainful employment and pleasure, and eventually one is oriented toward liberation in adherence to one's position in the varna system. Each person's position in the varna and their ashrama is considered integral in how they pursue the *purushartha*. The pravritti framework was (and still is) integral in the life of a savarna, as each life stage determines how engaged one is as a primary decision-maker of the household. As one approaches the *vanaprastha* stage, one is preparing to hand over familial responsibilities to the next generation.

Women, according to the pravritti dharmic traditions, are adjuncts who support, enable, and facilitate the religious life of the male householder.[4] The lives of savarna women, especially Brahmins and Kshatriyas, are thus inextricably intertwined with the supportive roles they play in the lives of their fathers, husbands, and sons, and to a lesser extent, their brothers. This ideal of a *pativrata* woman, the devoted wife, is an integral paradigm for aspirational behavior. This paternalistic leaning of the pravritti mode in the Vedic traditions forms the cornerstone of mainstream Indic cultures even today. The granularities of pravritti dharma are further elaborated in the Dharmashastras, such as Manava Dharmashastra. Ethics and moral codes in the dimension of pravritti dharma are not ubiquitous and universal; rather, they are situational and contextual. This means that sometimes *himsa* (violence) is ethical, if it means upholding one's dharma. Thus, in the Bhagavad Gita, Krishna tells Arjuna to fight the war, as it is the duty of a Kshatriya to uphold dharma, even when it means that he will be killing many of his kinfolk. This also rationalizes the subjugation of people, as each one has a place, a function, a role to play in the world. There are stories in the epics that demonstrate a certain fluidity between varnas, but as jaati becomes more rigid, social mobility becomes heavily restricted and confined to one's jaati identity.

Nivritti (turning away) dharma is the way of the renouncer, the one who is dedicated to spiritual goals through asceticism, a radical rejection of the attachments that arise from relationships, renouncing material pleasures and wealth accumulation beyond what is needed for basic survival. The ultimate goal of liberation from the cycles of birth and death is pursued with great fervor and rigor, and the values of self-discipline (*tapas*) supersede social harmony. In contrast to the worldly pursuit of the householder traditions of the pravritti dharma, nivritti espouses rigorous striving for moksha by practicing austerities, observing ahimsa, *brahmacharya* (celibacy), and equanimity at all times. Nivritti dharma "insists that true worth is to be measured by conduct, not by birth."[5] There is no regard for one's caste and class. One's gender, though, plays an important role. On the whole and across the caste spectrum, women have to face constraints placed upon them, from familial expectations to the broader societal concerns of clan and caste honor.

Patriarchy infuses both pravritti and nivritti dharma in distinct ways. Those who challenge these patriarchal norms within either of these frameworks are exceptional. Sulabha's assertion that she belongs to no one stems from the way of nivritti dharma. In the nivritti orientation, although there are a few references to *rishika*s (renunciate scholars of the Vedas) and *sanyasi*s (mendicants who relinquish all attachment, who beg for food and sometimes shelter as a commitment to their ideal of *vairagya* or nonattachment), women are seen as temptations that lead a serious yogi astray from their goals, especially in the later developments of hatha yoga (which we will discuss later). Women are also depicted as scholars, students, and partners, but only in relationship to the men who are fathers and husbands in the *vanaprastha* ashrama. Thus Sulabha, as a free-moving yogini is unique in her assertion of absolute independence.

Patriarchy as a Part of the Caste System

In a land where goddess worship is traced back to the Harappan civilization and even to this day is celebrated with great reverence and bhakti, where are the women, the femmes, in the lineages and traditions of yoga, and why does one have to dig through academic tomes to get to them? In other words, what is the historical context for the dominance of patriarchal narratives in the teachings of yoga?

Patriarchy, defined as a system of social structures and practices in which cis men are centered above all other genders, is one of the most ancient and tenacious social structures that has shaped, impacted, and dominated almost all cultures and civilizations through history. Patriarchy sets in as migrant, nomadic groups settle into land ownership, agriculture, and cultivation of crops. Prior to this, in nomadic hunting-gathering societies in central India in the Mesolithic period, it is likely that women participated in the hunt apart from all the important tasks of gathering. A recent study of cave paintings at Bhimbekta (ca. 5000 BCE) shows that there are multiple depictions of women hunting and fishing. There is a woman with a basket slung over her shoulder with two children in it, and she also carries an animal on her head. Another woman is dragging a deer by its antlers, and more women are engaged in fishing. The relative status of men and women in these paintings can be characterized as separate but equal.[6]

Agriculture necessitated clear boundaries of property ownership, both of land and of cattle. The impetus to protect one's property and ensure that wealth would be transferred to one's progeny shaped gender relationships. The pervasiveness of patriarchy was and continues to be the most important and almost invisible factor that shapes all realms, in all social-cultural-economic and spiritual dimensions. In this chapter, we will explore the foundations of the intersections of caste and gender and contextualize the emergence of archetypes of women that continue to impact South Asian culture and influence the practice and teachings of modern yoga.

Vedic women show up in a multitude of ways. While some of the verses are attributed to twenty-seven women sages, among them rishis (seers), *brahmacharini*s (Vedic ascetics), *brahmavadini*s (students of philosophy), and *sadyodvaha*s (scholars and teachers), they appear as notable mentions buried in the magnum opuses of the Vedas. The main corpus of the Vedic compositions, however, was centered around the Brahmin and Kshatriya men. The paucity of mentions or contributions of femme, women, and gender-expansive scholarship does not indicate a lack of contributions or active participation in spiritual life. It means they were not regarded as important enough to be remembered in the Vedic narrations of bards who were men.[7] Their stories are in relationship to the men as wives or daughters of sages; they are not the focus of the texts. Brahmin women are considered as ritual partners with their husbands, with clearly defined roles as *sahadharmini* (partner along with the man). Some star in poems on courtship and marriage as courtesans, wives, or mothers. Gargi, Maitreyi, and Lopamudra were regarded as learned scholars and philosophers. Women were also consorts of divine husbands, like Indrani, the wife of Indra, the king of the gods. The primal goddess Aditi, One Without Limits, is the one who gives birth to the whole of the cosmos, a representation of the creation of the universe from primordial energy.

While patriarchy embedded within the context of the varna system was expanding and gaining dominance, it still was not unilateral; there were philosophical, sociological, and ontological explorations in the Vedas. The Vedic literature also has multiple references to and detailed descriptions of diverse gender identities and queer sexualities in society and among deities. The *pums* (man) prakriti describes variations of the cis male, the *stri* (woman) prakriti describes the cis woman, and the *trittiya* prakriti elaborates on the "third gender" (what we refer to today as gender-expansive and intersex folks). There are over forty terms that describe the *trittiya* prakriti alone.[8] Some of the deities of the Vedic period are portrayed as having homosexual relationships, like Agni, the god of fire, with Soma, a deity of the moon. Per Vedic astrology, the nine planets are assigned genders: the Sun, Jupiter, and Mars were described with the masculine gender; the Moon, Venus, and Rahu are referred to as the feminine gender; and Mercury, Saturn, and Ketu are the third or neutral gender. While an analysis of gender and sexualities during the Vedic period is beyond the scope of this book, the elaborate descriptions of diverse genders and sexual orientations offer us an important clue about societal acceptance or at least acknowledgement of heterogeneity of gender expressions and experiences.

Around 100 CE the composition of Manava Dharmashastra (also known as Manu Smriti), one of several treatises on dharma, offered codes and laws for ethical conduct primarily addressed to Brahmin men. An adherence to these laws was positioned as a pathway for achieving moksha and sustaining *rta*, universal order. The text was also accretive, with layers added over centuries, which may explain contradictory statements such as "where women are revered, there the gods rejoice; but where they are not, no sacred rite bears any fruit," while also declaring, "a woman must never seek to live independently." As the Dharmashastras had Brahmin authors and commentators, there was a "bias in favor of those in authority."[9] Thus narratives around gender and caste that positioned cis-het Brahmin men as the ultimate religious and intellectual authority were amplified and codified through these texts and their subsequent translations. Manu Smriti elaborates on the status of women and gender minorities only in relationship to the men in their life; their sexual, economic, and intellectual freedoms were not important considerations.

The growing influence of Brahmanism also did not exclude alternate pathways to liberation beyond Vedic ritualism or sramanic asceticism. The earliest Tantra *sampradays* (traditions) emerged around the fifth century CE in Kashmir, Kamarupa (modern Orissa), and the Chola kingdom (modern Tamil Nadu). Tantra in many ways opposed some of the Vedic teachings about the illusory nature of reality and instead included all materiality as a manifestation of the sacred. In the beginning Tantra was a heterodox path open to all, regardless of caste and gender.

Tantra traverses Vedic, Buddhist, and Jain traditions. In contrast to the ascetic ideal, it seeks liberation through being engaged in the world. Some of the Tantra traditions refer to a caste subversion of sorts. In the seventh-century Shaivite text Svachchanda Tantra, the initiated discard their caste status, and are all united in the caste of Shiva. This nullification of caste upon one's initiation into the lineage does not mean there were no power differences; instead it created "several new hierarchical categories between the Tantric and the non-Tantric practitioners."[10]

In Tantra, no aspect of the body was considered taboo or impure, in contrast to the Brahmanic or ascetic approach, which viewed sexuality and the physical body in more stringent ways, as things to be mastered and controlled. This aspect of reverence for the body especially comes to life in Shakta Tantra, in which the *maithuna* rituals consider menstrual blood to be a potent fluid infused with sacred regenerative energies of Shakti.[11] The Brahmin orthodoxy of the Vedic times criticized such antinomian aspects of advanced Tantric practices, causing many to practice them in secret. By the seventh century, many householders started to practice Tantra, and many Tantra rituals gradually were absorbed into the mainstream. This also meant that the prevailing dynamics of caste, class, and gender were absorbed; for instance, many of the rituals were codified by Tantric Brahmins, mostly men. Many of the more antinomian practices were sanitized to make them more palatable for mostly savarna practitioners. Tantra is a vast field of study and practice, and it is beyond my expertise and the scope of the book. However, it is important for us to know about these contradictions and how subversive heterodox traditions like Tantra can also have an underlying dynamic of power and privilege.

Sex and Control

"Sexuality is the primary site of control of women by patriarchy."[12] Patriarchy frames women's sexuality as something to be feared and controlled, even as it holds in high esteem the centrality of a woman's role as a mother, the one who births the future. During Vedic times, it was recommended that marriage, procreation, and devotion to her husband be the focal points of a woman's life, articulating a *stri* dharma as the benchmark of her entire existence and the very essence of religiosity. In the pravritti dharma, *stri* dharma was considered as the axis for the spiritual and intellectual aspirations of the Brahmin woman. There were many Dharmashastras, but Manu Smriti stands out as the most emphatic and detailed in its articulations regarding the preservation of the varna system. The text emphasized how sexuality can be controlled through early child marriage: "A thirty-year-old man should marry a twelve-year-old girl who charms his heart, and a man of twenty-four an eight-year-old girl; and if duty is threatened, [he should marry] in haste."[13] A woman married at a young age had limitations on her autonomy in the choice of a spouse, her access to intellectual pursuits, and her behavior and relationships with other castes. Any sexual, spiritual, or intellectual transgression was punished with severity and violence, and the whole family of the woman who had transgressed would also face shame and dishonor.

Caste hierarchy and gender hierarchy are the organizational principles of the Brahmanical social order.[14] Control needed to be asserted over the

Brahmin women's sexuality in order to preserve the purity of the social order; thus, her chastity and loyalty to the men in her life was of preeminent value. This emphasis on ensuring that the Brahmin lineage stayed intact, untainted, and pure meant conversely that deviation in any way was regarded as impure or polluted. This purity-and-pollution framework has always undergirded the caste system. The control of savarna women's agency and sexuality was considered absolutely essential in order to preserve power and privilege embedded within the dominant varnas, specifically the Brahmins.

There was also a gradation of occupations as a "graded inequality"[15] of labor and laborers that placed the ritualism and intellectualism of the Brahmins at the very top and center. Radiating down and outward into the margins of villages were the avarna communities who performed the labor of farming, leatherwork, sanitation, and cremation. This perpetuated the inhumane observance of untouchability. The Dasa women of the conquered tribes, on the other hand, were made *dasis* or slaves of the Brahmin and Kshatriya women. Their sexuality was also controlled, but differently, to be used at the discretion of the savarnas who had undisputed rights to the bodies of untouchable women. By and large most women were sequestered to varying degrees, and gradually women's agency was increasingly curtailed during the Vedic period.

Varnasamkara, "the sexual intermingling of classes, [was] treated as the very worst state of affairs in society."[16] Manu details the order and hierarchy of women who are ideal wives for savarna men: A Brahmin, Kshatriya, or Vaishya man ideally is partnered with a woman from his own varna, and he may marry a Shudra woman as a second or third wife. These mixed-varna unions resulted in the creation of more jaatis. Rules governing sexual (or other kinds of) intermingling between the varnas became increasingly rigid as endogamy became the norm, which also meant stringent rules for controlling women's sexuality. *Varnasamkara* is described in the first chapter of the Gita, when Arjuna is utterly dejected and anguished at the prospect of killing his kinfolk. He tells Krishna why doing so would mean the advent of Kali Yuga, a period of darkness and evil. In chapter 1 of the Gita, he describes Kali Yuga thus:

> *If a clan is destroyed, its time honored traditions perish, and when traditions disappear, unrighteousness overtakes the entire clan.*
> *When unrighteousness prevails, O Varshneya,* * *the women of the clan become corrupted.*
> *When this happens, intermingling of classes results. (1:40–41)*

And he continues:

> *This intermingling of social classes creates unworthy clans, which destroys Varnas.*
> *Thus, the spirits of their ancestors fall, degraded, deprived of the ritual offerings of rice and water, and they are condemned to a hellish life. (1:42–43)[17]*

This description of miscegeny represents Kali Yuga, "the mythical dystopia, the ultimate degeneration and inversion of the moral order."[18] Here there is a clear articulation that Arjuna is reflecting on what society is grappling with: the value attributed to the safeguarding of parameters of *kula* (clan) and varna, and thus an emphasis on the sexual and moral activity of women. The framing of Kali Yuga as the depraved, self-indulgent, immoral, and unethical time period of human existence is rooted in a social and political context where the boundaries between varnas were drawn and also challenged. It is important to note how the meaning and implication of a word shifts through the centuries. Today, most people would use the term Kali Yuga to refer to dark and evil times when vice prevails.

Although the householder tradition of the pravritti dharma advocates an adherence to gendered roles and duties to maintain order, the ascetics from the nivritti dharma were also not exempt from gendered perspectives. In the fifteenth-century *Hatha Yoga Pradipika*, the influential hatha yoga text composed by Svatmarama, the directions in the teachings are clearly

---

* Another name for Krishna.

addressed to a man. For the one who has just commenced as a *sadhaka* (a spiritual aspirant), women are considered as temptations to be avoided, just as one would avoid other distractions and dangers:

> *Don't indulge in fires, women, or travel in the beginning.*
> *Goraksha says: Avoid bad people, fires, women, travel, early morning baths, fast-ing, etc., and actions that hurt the body. (1:61)[19]*

In the same text, women are addressed as yoginis who can draw up the semen of a man through the expert practice of the *vajroli* mudra:

> *She who preserves her seminal fluid by drawing upwards is indeed a yogini.*
> *She knows the past and the future, and surely moves in the sky. (3:102)[20]*

Traditional hatha yoga has its roots in Tantra, which considers the role of women as impediments for the beginner yogi and as partners for the more advanced. In the text, the yogi is the primary audience; the yogini appears as an aide in his goal of achieving samadhi (meditative absorption). As far as I know, there are no yoga texts addressed solely to femme/gender-expansive and women ascetics. This does not mean that there were no women or gender-expansive folks practicing asceticism. Sulabha's appearance in the Mahabharata shows us that it was not unheard of; Janaka is surprised by her youth and appearance, not that she is an ascetic. The lack of texts addressing women as primary students could be attributed to the orality of the teachings, and to the fact that the ones who got to scribe, codify, and organize were men.

Narratives of gender in the Puranas and the epics are informed by the archetypes in Vedic Brahmanism. They are rife with the stories of the Brah-min woman devoted to the men in her life, while the *dasi*s are either por-trayed as *rakshasi*s (female demons) or as sexually promiscuous women who need to be chastened in some way. In the Valmiki Ramayana, for instance, the main women characters in the epic are either a chaste loyal wife like Sita, a suffering mother like Kaushalya (Rama's mother), or an *asura* seductress like Shurpanaka, the sister of Ravana, who pays heavily for her bold invita-tions to Rama and Lakshmana. Although Valmiki refers to women ascetics, women's sexuality and desire are portrayed with suspicion and derision by those in power.

While the law books composed around the first century CE were a part of the religious and philosophical landscape, justice was carried out by a plethora of regional and communal laws.[21] The Manu Smriti gained prominence as a law book only after the British colonial administrators chose it for ease of administration and organization, as a device to categorize and govern the mind-boggling array of varying cultures and traditions prevalent in the Indian subcontinent. The project was to rule the Indians using their own laws, so the East India Company (the British monarchy's trading organization) sent a lawyer, William Jones, who translated the Manu Smriti circa 1794, thus rendering it more credible.

Caste also was included in the 1872 and 1881 censuses, which attempted to fundamentally classify people according to their varna as mentioned in ancient texts. Caste as a category of identification was thus institutionalized, and this mode of categorizing people persists to this day. The British elevation of the text to legal canon and the selective quotations from Manu Smriti by anticolonial Hindu nationalists such as Vinayak Damodar Savarkar, the architect of Hindutva, made this text a powerful influence in shaping independent India's legal and social ethos. Dr. Ambedkar, a staunch critic of the Manu Smriti, organized a burning of the text in 1927 in front of thousands, a day that Dalit communities all over the world celebrate as Manusmriti Dahan Divas (the Day of Burning of Manu Smriti).

Sanskrit as a Medium for Brahmanism

Vedic Sanskrit was the language of the elite. The local or the vernacular languages were a part of oral traditions that were often matrilineal and matriarchal in origin. They were not written down and hence were not accorded legitimacy. Therefore, a vast majority of rural traditions are dismissed as folklore because credibility is attributed to the written word, which was predominantly the domain of the cis-het Brahmin man. Everyday practitioners do not know about characters like Sulabha because written (and thus preserved) scholarship has been largely patriarchal, centering cis-heteronormative perspectives of Brahmin and European men. We study their understandings of the human body, discourses of human experiences, and aspirations stemming from their lived experiences. The definitions of creation, sustenance, and destruction come from texts and interpretations chosen from a Brahminical lens. What if Sulabha was as well-known as Arjuna? Both are figures from the epics, and many yoga practitioners know Arjuna because of his conversation on a battlefield that brought forth the teachings of the Bhagavad Gita. But not many know of Sulabha's discourse on gender, which is actually revolutionary. If her discourse were better known, how would that have expanded our understanding of gender? How would we receive femme agency? How would we think of a woman's capacity for intellectual and spiritual courage? These are questions worth pondering in the times we live in.

Vedas were composed in a formal "classical" Sanskrit, a language fiercely protected by Brahmin men. Millions revere Saṃskṛtam (not anglicized) or "perfectly constructed" Sanskrit as a divine language or *deva-vani* that is resonant with the sounds of the universe itself. The history of Sanskrit is highly controversial because there is a deep internalization of its sanctity, a reverential attribution of its ahistorical origin, and the notion that it had a supra-human source and was the mother of all languages in the subcontinent. As we have seen in the first chapter, the Indo-Aryans brought a form of archaic Sanskrit and used it for formal political announcements, conducting rituals, and composing the Vedas. The Harappans had different languages that evolved into Tamil, Kannada, Malayalam, and Telugu, spoken by people in the southern states of modern India. As trade and commerce proliferated, a script was developed for Sanskrit around 600–321 BCE to facilitate ease in transactions.[22] Thus Sanskrit became one of the first few languages in the region to be written down and preserved, lending it currency as the language of priests, scholars, and philosophers, which gave it an association with intellectual sophistication and spiritual gravitas.

Sanskrit is often extolled as a "pure" language, untouched and sacred, often associated with the Puranic goddess Saraswati, the deity of knowledge in the Hindu pantheon. However, this does not take into account the dynamism or complexity of Sanskrit's long history. Many of the non-Sanskrit languages and texts from the oral traditions made their way into the Sanskrit language.[23] This was not a unidirectional process; rather, it was a dynamic one in which Sanskrit texts and their corresponding ideals and deities seeped out in a process of vernacularization as the Sanskrit texts were retold and narrated in regional languages. Vernacularization took place concurrently with the process of Sanskritization, a term coined by sociologist M. N. Srinivas, defined as the process by which a caste-oppressed group or tribe changes its customs, rituals, ideology, and way of life in the direction of caste privilege. By changing certain habits, such as adopting practices around food and marriage, caste identification could change in a generation or two. Sanskritization meant not only the adoption of new customs and habits but also exposure to new ideas and values that have found frequent expression in the vast body of Sanskrit literature, sacred as well as secular. "Karma, dharma, samsara and moksha are examples of some of the most common Sanskritic theological ideas that occur frequently when people become Sanskritized."[24] This mobility was possible only for the middle tier of jaatis—not for Dalits or avarna folks.

Sanskrit was a medium, an ideological vehicle to communicate the ideals, experiences, aspirations, and perspectives of caste-privileged people, especially the Brahmins. It was also one of the devices for excluding people from access to resources. By forbidding people to defy the rules and boundaries between varnas and jaatis, and punishing those who did, class and caste were preserved, excluding multitudes from both material and spiritual spaces. The Manu Smriti's edicts give firm warnings of the dire fate that awaited if any once-born (avarna or Shudra) transgressed the boundaries:

> *If he mentions their name or caste maliciously, a red-hot iron nail ten-fingers long should be thrust into his mouth. (8:271)*[25]
> *If he arrogantly gives instructions on the Law to a Brahmin, the king should pour hot oil into his mouth and ears. (8:272)*[26]

These *shloka*s indicate that the language and even the names of Brahmins were not allowed to be mentioned out loud by caste-oppressed folks. Vedic gods also have varnas assigned to them. Agni and Varuna are Brahmins and Indra is a Kshatriya, but there are no Shudra gods in the Vedas.[27] There was a clear boundary drawn between who was considered worthy of being deemed as a divine being, who could access the teachings of the Vedas, and who couldn't. These boundaries, amorphous at first, were firmed up through centuries. The conflicts between the varnas were reflected in some of the stories in the epics, such as the story of Ekalavya in the Mahabharata. Ekalavya, the scion of a tribal community, approached Dronacharya, the mighty guru of the Pandavas and the Kauravas. Drona refused to teach Ekalavya because he was from a tribal community and not from the princely or the scholarly class. Ekalavya went ahead with his training, keeping a clay statue of Dronacharya, and went on to become the best archer in the land, surpassing Arjuna's prowess. When Drona witnessed his expertise, he demanded a sacrifice of Ekalavya's right thumb as a guru *dakshina*, the gift one paid to one's teacher at the end of one's education, thus ensuring he never surpassed Arjuna as the most proficient archer in the land.

Women were also not allowed access to classical Sanskrit. The paucity of women's writing in classical Sanskrit is due to it being the language of religion and courtly art, used only by dominant-caste men.[28] There are a few stanzas from Vijjakka, the Buddhist scholar from modern Karnataka, dated around 650 CE. Though little is known of Vijjakka, her verses begin thus: "Without knowing about me, Vijjakka, dark, like the petal of the blue lotus, / That the poet Dandin said that the Goddess of learning was all-white."[29] In these two poignant verses, Vijjakka seems to be gently admonishing the Puranic period's elite worship of Saraswati, the goddess of learning, which excluded people like her.

The earliest women's writing is in Pali: the Therigatha or Songs of the Buddhist Nuns, composed around 600 BCE. Although Buddha was far more egalitarian with regard to class and caste, he was wary of allowing women in the sangha. The story of Buddha's foster mother, Mahapajapathi Gotami, highlights the patriarchal ideologies of the early Buddhist period. Gotami, longing to be ordained as a nun, braved long distances to beseech the Buddha to allow her into the sangha. When Buddha demurred, one of his young disciples, Ananda, intervened on her behalf, saying that according to the tenets of his teachings, everyone can gain spiritual emancipation. Buddha finally agreed, but only after laying down eight inviolable laws that any *theri* (nun) would have to obey. For example, no *theri* was allowed to defy or reproach a *thera* (monk), but a *thera* could discipline a *theri* at any time. After a two-year probationary period, the *theri* had to be confirmed by both the *theri*s and the *thera*s, whereas a *thera* only had to seek confirmation from the male order.

The Therigatha were first sung by the nuns as they wandered from village to village; later they were written down. They are filled with tales of spiritual longing and accounts of how Buddha showed them the way to enlightenment, a release from the cycle of birth and death. In one song, a *theri* named Mutta exults at a release from drudgery as she also seeks liberation from rebirth and death:

> *Free from three petty things—*
> *From mortar, from pestle and from my twisted lord,*
> *And all that has held me down*
> *Is hurled away.*[30]

It is moving to know of these ancestral voices of people living in times so different from ours and yet confronted with the same struggles of seeking agency and autonomy. Heterodox traditions like Buddhism, Jainism, Tantra, and later the Bhakti movement challenged the stratifications of orthodoxy; still, men mostly held the locus of power and the seat of the teacher. Thus people like Mutta, who persisted in their path toward liberation in the face of insurmountable systemic and personal obstacles, are an effulgent light for us today.

Gender Fluidity in Ancient Narratives

It is not female nor is it male nor is it neuter
It is joined with whatever body it takes.

—SHVETASHVATARA UPANISHAD 5.10[31]

The Upanishads eloquently explore the nature of the Atma. One of the most integral teachings of the Upanishads is that we are consciousness and that form, matter, and identity are ever-changing. Sulabha's dialectic exchange with Janaka is rooted in the Upanishadic teaching that the perennial essence of the Atma is the only constant and that everything else is transitory. Yoga is the practice of self-realization through which we realize that we are not our body, not our emotions, not our thoughts, and yet we identify with samsara or the world of sensory perception. The composers of the Upanishads use lyrical imagery and metaphors of union to describe the dynamics of fusion and liberation of matter and spirit. Their language communicates paradigms that delve into the nature of consciousness. We cannot easily think or articulate beyond the limits of language.[32] Language is a factor in shaping our inner world; how we perceive the world is communicated through language, which gives form to what we consider as truths. These "truths" then form our institutions and systems. When it comes to the construction of gender, language plays a pivotal and complex role. Sanskrit has three genders—masculine, feminine, and neutral—so English translations have a limitation.

Samkhya philosophy informs influential texts like Patanjali's Yoga Sutras and the Bhagavad Gita, in which there are ontological investigations (theories of being) into the dichotomies of purusa (consciousness) and prakriti (manifest, primordial nature). Samkhya offers a gendered view of the universe in metaphorical and allegorical language. Prakriti is gendered female, and purusa is gendered male. All beings have both prakriti and purusa, and this is not related to one's gender identification in real life; and yet, these concepts and their associated values have been internalized as absolute truths and binaries. Prakriti, as mutable, ever-changing, sensory, is contrasted with masculine-gendered purusa, the eternal witness, immutable, ascetic in essence. Prakriti is materiality; purusa is inactive, incapable of creative activity.

In the classical text Samkhya Karika, the term "Shakti" is used to designate "the capacity of prakriti to unfold."[33] Prakriti is the one who entices, who is the material essence of samsara; the sensory world thus represents pleasure and enjoyment, as well as lust and uninhibited chaos. Prakriti is the *kshetra* (field), rife with multiplicities, and purusa is the *kshetrajna*, the knower of the field.

The epics and the Puranas weave narratives around how ascetics are tempted to stray from their goal of self-realization because of prakriti, both within their own selves and also embodied as *apsaras* (celestial nymphs) who are portrayed as skilled temptresses. Emancipation—spiritual, political, and economic—is perceived as a goal that can be within the reach of the masculine, whereas the feminine is regarded as one who can support the man and yet has to strive harder to overcome an innate restlessness, solely due to the attributes of gender. In this way the gendered values of prakriti as ever-changing and thus fickle, and purusa as ever-present and thus stable, are projected onto human expression.

In the following passage from the Rig Veda, a declaration of immanence by the goddess Vak shows that goddesses are not merely embodiments of nature; they are nature and spirit both:

> *I am queen, gatherer of riches, knowing, the first among those worthy of being*
> *honored.*
> *I am she, having many stations and much bestowing, whom the gods have*
> *distributed in many places.*
> *I make him a Brahmin, I make him a seer (rishi), I make him wise.*
> *My yoni (womb/origin) is within the waters (ap) in the ocean (samudra).*
> *Beyond heaven, beyond the earth, so great have I*
> *Become through my grandeur. (10.125)*[34]

The epics include characters like Shikhandi, the brave transgender warrior in the Mahabharata, who kills the indefatigable Bhishma, the grand old commander of the Kauravas. Arjuna transforms into Brihannala, a trans femme dance teacher, during their exile in the forest. There is a tale in the same great epic of a king who gets pregnant. In the story, Yuvanashva, the prince of Vallabhi, is unable to father children, so his mother, Shilavati, will not allow him to be the king. He drinks a potion intended for his wives and then becomes pregnant himself. The birth of his son, Mandhata, leads Yuvanashva to question his gender identity, and he longs for his child to call him "mother."

The portrayals of women are complex. They are fiery queens of powerful husbands, and some even have five husbands, like Draupadi in the Mahabharata. Some are depicted as the dutiful wife who accompanies her banished prince to a forest and lives in great penury, like Sita of the other great epic, Ramayana. She is a sensual courtesan, an esoteric goddess, and everything in between, both pious and tempting of a Brahmin man's piety. There is complexities and contradictions galore in the literature, reflecting a society undergoing rapid growth and urbanization. These characters point to a time when patriarchy and gender were being questioned, when the ascetic ideal of renunciation (nivritti dharma) was challenged by the path of the householder (pravritti dharma).

Gender fluidity is narrated in the stories of Krishna and Shiva. The *ardhanareeshwara* (*ardha*: half; *naree*: woman; Ishwara: Shiva) form is the manifestation of the fluidity between purusa and prakriti, embodied as Shiva and Shakti. Krishna changes gender to become the dancer Mohini, an enchantress to divert the *asuras*' attention away from *amrita*, the elixir for immortality. The *asuras* get drawn into Mohini's celestial dance and temporarily forget about the *amrita*, and thus Mohini saves the societal order. The shape-shifting/gender-fluid, nonbinary Mohini is revered as a deity of the heart (*ishta-devata*) for many *hijra* (transgender/intersex folks in India). On a personal note, one of my ancestral temples in Goa is dedicated to Mahalasa, another name for Mohini!

There is also a profusion of stories of gender fluidity in the legends and tales of non-Vedantic or Puranic sources. In the Guntur district of Andhra Pradesh (a state in south India), there is a worship of the *chanti lingam* (*lingam* of the breast). The story goes that a sage named Oduyanambi had taken a vow that he would worship the *lingam* every three hours. However, after a night with his beloved, he lost all track of time and forgot his vow. Stricken with the possibility of breaking his pledge, he was frantic until his eyes fell on the left breast of his beloved. Filled with devotion, it appeared to him as the *lingam*, so he lovingly applied sandalwood paste to it and made offerings of betel leaves. From that day on, the village celebrated with the worship of the *chanti lingam.*[35]

Even with all these explorations in gender and sexuality, the dominant narratives in the Puranas center around cis Brahmin men as the ones who have the spiritual technology for moksha, and Kshatriya warriors as the patrons and the guardians of property and material wealth. The philosophical and spiritual contributions of all other teachers get buried deep due to multiple interlinked factors such as patriarchy, the rise and concretization of the caste system, the domination of the Brahmins (scholars) in all spiritual matters, and, of course, imperialism and colonization. Most of the yoga texts from the Bhagavad Gita (second or first century BCE) to the *Hatha Yoga Pradipika* (fifteenth century CE) have verses that point to the portrayal of women as those who pose obstacles for the dedicated yogi. There is a gender bias because the composers (or at least whose compositions were preserved through writing) and the subsequent translators, commentators, teachers, and proponents of these seminal texts were Brahmin men. These gender binaries are manifested in all the realms of yoga (and beyond), from cuing in a modern yoga class to erasures of gender-expansive folks as leaders and teachers. Stories like those of Sulabha, Shikhandi, and Mohini, mythical figures who transgressed and challenged dichotomies and binaries, need to be more prominent within mainstream yoga studies rather than being relegated to scholarly dissertations or esoteric literature.

Key Takeaways

Radical Debates as Resistance

Sulabha's debate with Janaka is one of many in the Upanishads. Two debates with the revered seer Yajnavalka are relevant to our discussion. In the Brihadaranyaka Upanishad, the scholar Gargi steps forward to challenge Yajnavalka. She declares to all gathered that she will pose two questions, and if he answers the two to her satisfaction, that in itself is enough for others to bow down to him as the most venerable scholar. The other debate, between Yajnavalka and his wife, Maitreyi, is referred to by many Indians even today to discuss the relationship between material wealth and moksha. While debates and conversation were often used as rhetorical devices in Upanishadic and Puranic literature to advance theses or expound upon a particular concept, they also reveal that there were a few notable women scholars at the time who were unafraid and "immodest" enough to go into a room full of men. The debates were formal in format and rigorous in the scale and depth of topics and interrogations they pursued, delving into the complexities of human existence and the nature of God and the universe. The sharpest questionings come from women interlocutors.[36] While feminism is more of a modern movement, if we dig deeper into ancient texts, we will find powerful voices that have been silenced and/or forgotten. We find that the issues of gender and power that dominate the current sociopolitical environment were prevalent during those times too.

Sulabha's assertion that she is equally capable of achieving moksha draws from the underlying notion of the oneness of all of creation and that one's physical denomination of sex is acquired and can change during one's lifetime. She reiterates that gender is a social construct. (Since I refer to Ruth Vanita's scholarship on this, I do not know the emic language from the original verses in the Mahabharata.) Gender fluidity was and still is a very controversial concept for many. Although Sulabha's debate pertains to self-realization or moksha, her rhetoric of ownership of herself as belonging to no other and of having the same potential as the king to achieve spiritual transformation is pertinent even now, as the modern world still struggles with this concept of equity and access to resources across genders. Sulabha's choice to remain single and pursue a path of enlightenment is unique, especially during her time, when women depended on men and women's spiritual prowess was connected to devotion and piety in relationship to men, forging a hierarchy that placed the cis man at the top. If we unearthed more of the sheer brilliance of the unfettered ancient women/femme and nonbinary wisdom holders and teachers, imagine how that would light us up in our despair at the state of the world today, where gender disparity shows up in all realms: reproductive justice, trans liberation, and equal access to safety, education, health care, and employment.

Yet another myth is that it was the West who emancipated women in yoga. Although it is true that Indra Devi, originally named Eugenia Petersen, a tenacious Latvian-born teacher, was the first woman student of Sri Krishnamacharya in the Mysore palace, it is not accurate to state that she was the first woman to practice yoga or even bring it to the West. She popularized the practice in the United States, but women and nonbinary practitioners have practiced and taught some form of yoga throughout the ages. Whether as portrayals of the scholarly *rishikas* such as Sulabha and Gargi from ancient times, or as the women in Tantra traditions called yoginis, believed to have occult and supernatural powers, women were always a part of yogic traditions. We know of these women through literature, poetry, art, and architecture. For instance, the ninth-century Chausath Yogini temple in Odisha, India (also known as the "sixty-four yogini temple") features idols of goddess figures standing on various animals or *vahana*s (vehicles) considered to be embodiments of Shakti. There are also paintings from the seventeenth century depicting female ascetics from the Nath tradition. All of these point to some of the yogic lineages having practitioners from different lived experiences.

Although gender archetypes from the Vedic period have survived to influence the social, political, economic, and cultural ethos of the entire subcontinent, it is important to be wary of broad generalizations in the presence of variations of class, caste, region, and language. We need to take careful account of the "spatial, historical, and communitarian specificity of a woman in order to make an academically intelligible statement."[37] Patriarchy impacts different people differently; thus, Shudra, Dalit, and Adivasi women have had to resist the harm of Brahmanism and patriarchy differently from caste-privileged women.

An exemplary example of caste and feminist resistance is Savitribai Phule, a nineteenth-century educator and the wife of Jyotirao Phule, a social activist and anticaste leader. She, like most women of her time, was not allowed to be educated. Public education, which was mostly run by Christian missionaries, only allowed the rich elite and/or Brahmin boys. Jyotirao encouraged Savitribai to study at home and attend one of the few institutions run by an American missionary in Ahmednagar that admitted women and people from all castes, where she completed her training as a teacher. She met Fatima Sheikh, a Muslim woman who, like her, faced innumerable societal barriers to getting an education. Their friendship, camaraderie, and sisterhood define the core values of what we call intersectional feminism today.[38] The Phules were not Dalits but were from a caste-oppressed community, and both worked tirelessly to open high-quality educational institutions that welcomed students from all caste backgrounds. They also challenged other misogynist norms, like female infanticide, and they encouraged marriage between different castes. She is regarded as a feminist icon today, but during her lifetime she braved unimaginable and heinous taunting, with stones and dung thrown at her while she walked to school.

Even though there have been luminaries throughout history like Savitribai Phule, who resisted both Brahmanism and patriarchy, in the twenty-first century the *pativrata* ideal still persists in all domains. This ideal is enacted through legislation such as section 375 of the Indian Penal Code, which does not consider marital rape to be a criminal offense, and imposition of paternalistic methods of policing women's agency and sexuality. The "anti-Romeo" squads that are often sanctioned by state machinery harass and arrest consenting adults in intercaste and interreligious relationships. Even though honor killings—in which the *izzat* (honor) of the family depends upon the virginity/chastity of the woman—are vastly underreported, a study shows that nearly five thousand women and girls are killed annually, and one third of them come from India and Pakistan.[39] Any infraction or defiance in the form of a premarital relationship, marriage outside the caste/religion, marriage within the same clan (*gotra*), relationship against the consent of the parents, adultery, or divorce is duly punished.[40] According to Dalit rights activist Thenmozhi Soundararajan, "The average age of death for Dalit women is thirty-nine," and "a crime against a Dalit happens every eighteen minutes."[41] In acknowledgement of my privilege as a caste-privileged savarna woman who lives in the United States, I share only some of these statistics, not to co-opt the sufferings but to highlight how relationships of caste, class, and gender are still deeply influenced by the misogynistic tenets of texts like the Manu Smriti that have violently harmed so many and continue to harm millions today.

Patriarchy and misogyny impact different people differently, manifesting in unique and specific ways. There are patriarchal and misogynistic themes and tenets as well as movements of feminist resistance in every major religion, from Islam and Christianity to Buddhism, Judaism, and Jainism. In the United States they exist in every dimension, from pay parity across gender and race lines to reproductive justice to inequities in health care, especially for Black, Indigenous, and trans women. I have highlighted only some of the threads of texts related to yoga and how they continue to shape different communities. Thus, stories from the past continue to be present in many ways.

Sanskrit as an Ancestral Language

Sanskrit is widely acknowledged as the "language of yoga." From asana names to "yoga" texts, Sanskrit is considered the de facto medium for transmission of spiritual teachings. However, it was and is not accessible to Shudras, Dalits, Bahujan, and other caste-oppressed folks who were violently prevented from even mentioning Brahmin names. Thus, emphasizing the narrative that one has to study Sanskrit in order to practice or teach yoga does not take into account the trauma experienced by folks who could not study or chant due to caste.

Sanskrit is not the only language of yoga; it is *one* of the languages of yoga. Sanskrit is an ancestral language with a long and complex history of caste oppression. It is also a language that transmits lyrical teachings of liberation, love, transcendence, human longing for and wondering about something more sublime and connection to the divine. As a yoga community, in solidarity with caste-marginalized folks who have experienced intergenerational harm and violence, we can invite each person to have agency and choice in the use of Sanskrit. Cultivating spaces that hold complexity and multiplicities of perspectives, practices, cultures, and languages is important to the intentional deconstruction of casteist power hierarchies in yoga and beyond. As yoga practitioners, we can democratize the study of texts from non-Sanskrit sources, thereby also inviting different worldviews and lived experiences. This is the dire need of the times, as we are deeply enmeshed in polarities of thought, opinion, and positionalities.

Building relationships with folks who have been and still are wary of coming to yoga because of past and ongoing caste discrimination is also crucial. The teachings of yoga can help us hold tension and discomfort and can nourish and support our nervous system so we are more responsive to rise to the challenge of disrupting long-held belief systems that are internalized as absolute truths.

Interrogate Narratives Around Purity and Pollution

Essentializing yoga as an unchanging tradition does a disservice to contemporary practitioners, as it does not represent the entirety of the yoga tapestry. This notion that yoga is pristine and should not be criticized comes partly from deeply held *samskaras* (in this context, defined broadly as deeply internalized impressions and patterns of thought) holding that we have to preserve this mythical purity of a thing, of a practice, of a tradition, of a culture, of a language, of a relationship. But this belief is not rooted in the historical realities of complications and paradoxes; it stems from our cultural conditioning about perfectionism and purity. Human beings are messy. We aspire to clarity, justice, love, and healing, and yet we vie with each other for power and cause harm. Yoga is not immune to the quagmire of the human experience. The stories in yoga are testament that there were struggles both within and without when a *sadhaka* or *sadhaki* (spiritual aspirant) went through trials and tribulations to achieve moksha. The social strife created by caste, gender, religion, class, and race was constructed by the same people who also aspired to spiritual liberation (moksha). Thus, nothing is really completely pure; yet we still seek this fantasy. We do so because of the narratives around purity that are rooted in hierarchical definitions of what is pure and impure.

In Sanskrit and many regional Indian languages, *shuddh* and *ashuddh* mean pure and impure, respectively. These terms are used widely and almost colloquially to denote the purity and hence quality of something. Many commercials that sell "Indian ghee" proclaim that they are selling *shuddh* desi ghee. "Pure vegetarian" is a phrase commonly used to identify restaurants that serve vegetarian food, and people who eat vegetarian thus are "pure vegetarians." The notions of purity and pollution pervade many aspects of ayurveda, yoga, diet, and other cultural and social practices. These narratives are extended toward every aspect of a person's life, from diet to occupation choices, and are rooted in Brahmanism. Taken to the extremes, this has harmed many and continues to harm millions of folks impacted by caste marginalization. The prejudice against nonvegetarian castes and religions is prevalent in the diaspora, too. Many vegetarian folks do not even eat in homes that cook meat (like mine). Foods are classified according to what is considered pure and associated with light, clarity, and spiritual superiority, whereas the opposite is impure or polluted, with corresponding associations of darkness and lethargy. As discerning yoga practitioners, we can be more conscious of how these values are historically and socially constructed.

Expand Inquiries of Brahmanical Patriarchy in Yoga History

While there is some knowledge of *rishika*s like Gargi or Maitreyi or the later bhakti practitioners, there is inadequate interrogation of the truth that most yoga gurus, ancient and modern, are and have been cis men. It is thus an irony that the modern yoga studio or a yoga class has mostly cis women attendees. While there are perhaps feminist perspectives and practitioners delving into the Yoga Sutras or even the *Hatha Yoga Pradipika*, the authors of those texts were men. So the question is: Are there texts or compositions that we do not or cannot learn from because they were erased or were never written down for posterity? We may never know. It is worth mulling over and continuing to seek sources that provide answers to these questions. There is a dire need to challenge misogynistic themes in yoga teachings. The texts come from a world that looks and sounds different from our own. Teachings around the intersections of caste and gender need to be studied for what they are: reflections of the time of their composition that nevertheless impact modern social and political systems.

Holding multiplicities, the both/and of a situation—a practice, a culture, a language, a relationship—is imperative as we find ourselves increasingly involved in polarities of thought, opinion, and positionalities. Brahmanical patriarchy has also been challenged and countered in disruptive uprisings throughout history by bhakti: outpourings of devotion to and love for the sacred that spontaneously burst forth in a poet's ballads, a sculptor's chisel, a potter's wheel, a weaver's tapestry, a milkmaid's song, and a queen's defiance. This devotion, this passionate fire of longing, a yearning for the sublime, this innate knowing of one's connection with the profound persists as living traditions even today. Mostly practiced and experienced by women and folks from caste-oppressed communities, bhakti revolutionized orthodoxies across time, imagination and space, manifesting sacred resistance.

Summary

Sulabha's debate with Janaka elucidates a key Upanishadic teaching of the nature of Atma: that it is untouched by social constructs of gender and caste. As Brahmanical orthodoxy spreads, gender too becomes stratified, with the domains of power mostly occupied by Brahmin and Kshatriya men. Although there are heterodox traditions of Buddhism, Jainism, Tantra, and bhakti, patriarchy seeps through in all aspects of culture, including the teachings of yoga. It is therefore important for modern yoga practitioners to be discerning of the internalization of some of these intergenerational norms and values.

May Sulabha's fierce admonition to Janaka serve as an invitation for us to heed that we are spiritual beings having a physical experience.

May we remember her song in our quest for liberation from suffering—a quest that is universal and should not be defined or limited by our gender or any other factor.

- What are some of the systemic obstacles that prevent us from expanding our capacity to hold the both/and of ourselves, each other, and the world?

- How have the narratives of purity and pollution shaped and impacted your yoga practice? What are some words that point to this framework in your daily life, off the mat?

- How can we cocreate intentional communities to hold and process complexities?

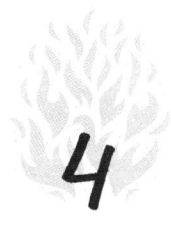

4

THE DANCE OF RADHA

She was the Poornima moon in a sea of stars.
She bit his lip, he tugged her hair.
The doe looked on, the flower blushed.
Her jhumka *(earring) gleamed in the silver light.*
Her feet, his hands, his caress, her sigh
Echoes in the jasmine grove, a heady union
The warm embrace of earth and spirit
Radha, his lover,
Radha, his Radha,
Radhe, Radha, Radhika
His muse, his beloved, his teacher.

Radha and Krishna, they were inseparable. She taught him everything.
She knew everything; the winding ways of the river Yamuna from the heavens
onto the Earth, how the sacred waters nourished the wise, old rishis in their ash-
rams along the banks, how to make special medicine from the golden lotus to
mend broken bones, and precisely when the kohda *tree sheds its magical bark.*
She studied the clouds and knew when it would rain, she could feel the change
of the seasons in her bones.

She knew every one of them, they knew her, Vrindavan's pride and joy, the
nine hundred thousand cows of Nanda, his foster father. There was Surbhi with
her gray-brown eyes, playfully nuzzling the little one, Manoratha. There was
Pingala, the one who always lingered behind. She taught him their names, and

how to speak to them, to listen to their calls, to get them together before dusk fell. She carved the bansuri, *a flute from bamboo, taught Krishna melody and rhythm and showed him the wild ecstasy of dance. Dance they did, wildly, joyfully, freely weaving in and out, their raucous laughter ringing out in the forests, mingling with the songs of the nightingale; long hair free to the wind, hands raised to the skies, then clasping with one another, round and round they went in an intricate dance until they had to stop for a breath, then they started all over again.*

She was bold, this Radha, unflinchingly staring down a tiger one day, dancing on the head of the crocodile the next, as if to say, O Nature, I am You, You are Me, We are One! She taught him how to ride horses, not just one, but many at a time, and rein them in at his will. She taught him the laws of the jungle, leading him by his hand when all were asleep, to witness how the tigress guards her young, even if that means she has to kill, how the flesh of the slain deer feeds the leopards, how everything perishes, changes forms and comes back to life. She educated him on the power of the breath and how the breath shapes one's thoughts, she shared the mantra of the Gayatri and revealed the eternal Truths known only to the Brahmarishis. It was as if she knew his destiny.

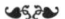

Tracing Radha

Radha and I go back a long way. The above *katha* is my version of the story of Radha and Krishna. I take this liberty for three main reasons. First, Radha is an embodiment of bhakti. She is a poet's muse, born of imagination and prayer, brought to life in dance and song, forever the eternal lover. Second, a subversion of their story is also an ode to her defiant and persistent subversiveness. She was a humble *gopika*, a milkmaid, a married older woman; yet bards and poets have sung paeans about her intense and passionate relationship with Krishna in the gardens of Vrindavan. They usually met surreptitiously, in the dark, in a lush forest, away from prying eyes.

The third reason is personal. As a young dancer, I portrayed the role of Radha, so this connection feels real and embodied to me. I would often grapple with how I as a young teen could even depict the depths of her emotionality. She is the embodiment of grace and fire. To enact that *bhava* (emotion) with integrity, with as much honesty as a teen could muster, was both an aspiration and an inspiration. I would often wonder: How it would be to love so deeply? How would it be to be loved so deeply? How would it be to know that such love has no other ambition but the sheer experience of it? I was intrigued by the stories of her deep, wanton love for Krishna, of her fierce pride and his preference for her above all else. It made me hunger to know more about her and her enigmatic story. What attracted the hero Krishna, the cynosure of everyone's attention, to her? What happened to her after he left her to go accomplish all that he did and all that he became, an influential chieftain of the Yadava clan, a diplomat and a philosopher on a battlefield, whose words still reverberate today?

Radha's story is steeped in folklore and the Puranas. She traverses different worlds with ease. Her depictions range from the inherent creativity that art gives humanity to the more structured constructs of religion. This breadth of range is not accorded to many depictions of femme figures. Saraswati and Lakshmi are pristinely presented goddesses who are never depicted in passionate, romantic relationships with their divine consorts. While there are stories of Parvati with Shiva, they are enveloped in a mystical and mythical chassis. Radha is earthy and relatable; she cajoles her lover and makes demands of him, and she expresses insecurities when he leaves her, like most humans would. She is revealed in songs and dance as a folk heroine and is worshipped as an incarnation of Lakshmi. For these reasons, her story is ideal for unraveling the dynamics and complexities of integration and appropriation of tribal icons into a pantheistic scaffolding.

Radha is also a study of the juicy complexities of contradictions. Her identity is as a beloved of Krishna, yet it is her choice to meet him; there is no other societal compunction. She is bold and defiant, yet she is also vulnerable and longs for their union when they are apart. Radha (or Radhika as she is also known) is the quintessential beloved in many a tale and lore, not a real woman of flesh and blood; yet most who have heard of Krishna have also heard of her. She is a mystery; there is not much detail of her home life. Was she a figment of some ancient imagination? Was she fashioned after a lost love? Was she created from a collective longing for an intimate, personal, human relationship with the divine? Was she the personification of a bard's admiration for the rebellious abandonment of guilt or shame about rejoicing in pleasure? We only know what we have been told through poetry, prose, architecture, and music. There is more to her than this love for Krishna. She also holds a mirror to other important tales of the times. She is an emblem, a symbol. Where does her story begin, and does it have an ending? Who was she? Was she a real person? If she was not a real person, what inspired her creation?

Radha is alive in a practitioner's bhakti consciousness, worshiped as a goddess in all kinds of places and ways, from magnificent marble temples to humble home altars to makeshift street shrines made of stone and straw. She is bedecked and bejeweled, standing tall with a beauteous smile alongside her beloved Krishna as if exulting in her good fortune to be in such close proximity with the one she loves—eternal lovers indeed! Their names are even said together: Radhakrishna is Krishna. Even if her figure is not next to him, she still is present, very much so, in our hearts and imagination, in our bhakti. This is her triumph. But the questions remain: What was the trajectory of her portrayal? She is first mentioned as a milkmaid from a community of herders; then she is hailed as a Puranic goddess. What can we glean from this transition about how symbols and icons are created, developed, integrated, and appropriated?

Radha was born of the ahistorical collective consciousness of religion and culture.[1] She was a heroine of popular culture who was not mentioned in Sanskrit texts such as the Vedas or Upanishads, and not even in the Mahabharata, where Krishna played such a pivotal role. Rather, she emerges from the periphery of Brahmanical culture, not the center.[2] The earliest mention of Radha comes in the Gatha Saptasati, a collection of seven hundred verses dated around the second century CE. This anthology of poems compiled by Hala, a king from the first century, is themed around the ups and downs of complicated human relationships. It has all the proclivities and shades of love and longing. The poems refer to village life, community gatherings around festivals, secret meetings with lovers, and prayers to gods and goddesses. In this secular, romantic, and bucolic milieu, Radha makes her appearance:

> *O Krishna, by the puff of breath from your mouth, as you blow the dust from*
> *Radha's face,*
> *You take away the glories of other milkmaids.*[3]

Radha may not be the central protagonist in the early texts, yet her presence commands a certain attention because her character feels real and compelling. Some of the texts are composed in lands far away from each other, in faiths that sometimes diverge, yet her core story tugs at the same chords of passion and emotion. Many scholars believe that the heroine Nappinnai of the fifth-century Tamil epic Silappadikaram is Radha.[4] There are also references to Radha in Jain drama and literature. However, it took a few centuries for Radha to surface in Puranic literature. In the ninth-century Vaishnavite Sanskrit composition Bhagavat Purana, there is a mention of Anyaradhita or the conciliated one, an appellation designating someone who is singled out for special favors, rather than a proper noun naming an individual.[5] The Bhagavat Purana was composed deep in Tamil country, in the south of ancient India, not in Braj or Mathura, the two places that are most closely associated with Krishna's roots. This text is centered around telling stories about the loving worship (bhakti) of Krishna that integrates divergent schools of philosophy.

The Bhakti movement, a cultural reform movement focused on bhakti as an approach to salvation, emerged in south India with the poet-saints, a diverse collection of religious and socially concerned teachers, in the worship of Shiva with the Nayanars (fifth to tenth centuries CE) and the worship of Vishnu with the Alvars (sixth to ninth centuries CE). Some scholars believe that the stories of Radha were also inspired by stories of Andal, the Alvar saint who professed devotion to Krishna at a young age.[6] This region was also important for generating a corpus of literature and secular poetry (100 BC–250 CE), including some of the oldest extant poems written by women in India. A total of 154 of the 2,381 *sangam* poems have "women's signatures."[7] The poems do not have many Sanskrit words and little in the way of Indo-Aryan mythology, suggesting that the regions had yet to be shaped by Vedic Brahmanism. Thus, the south of medieval India—which was less influenced by the more patriarchal structures of Indo-Aryan culture—had many folk heroines who may have not only inspired the story of Radha but also kept it alive and vibrant in people's collective consciousness.

Over the ensuing centuries, Radha's portrayal changes from a cowherdess of modest means to a goddess. This transition is not linear, even though she is referred to as a *devi* in the Sanskrit texts; she weaves in and out of regional dramas, folk songs, paintings, and erotic poetry. She is mentioned in the Devi Bhagavata, the Brahma Vaivarta, and the Padma Purana,[8] in which she is referred to as an incarnation of Lakshmi and is thus worshiped as an avatar of the goddess of prosperity. Even with these multitudinous portrayals and mentions, she is still not the main protagonist; rather she is a notable mention who over time became pedestalized as a goddess. She comes into her own as a full-blooded, open-hearted, wildly sensual human heroine or *nayika* of her beloved dark lord, Krishna (Krishna is often portrayed with dark skin, almost a deep blue), in the twelfth-century Bhakti poet-saint Jayadeva's erotic, dramatic, and lyrical masterpiece *Gita Govinda*.

"Radha, you take him home!"
They leave at Nanda's order
Passing trees in thickets on the way,
Until secret passions of Radha and Madhava
Triumph on the Jamuna riverbank.[9]

We meet Radha in the very first verse of *Gita Govinda*, not as Krishna's spouse, lover, or devotee. She is an independent older woman who is asked by Nanda, Krishna's foster father, to take Madhava (another name for Krishna) home through the forests—a meeting that leads to them becoming lovers. The very first scene set by Jayadeva, with poetic imagery of the clouds and dark, thick trees that loom large evokes palpable excitement and heightened sensory awareness. The first meeting ends in passionate lovemaking between Krishna and Radha. The reader/audience is then taken through a deeply emotional, mystical, wildly erotic, lyrical story of an episode in their relationship. Radha is forlorn when Krishna leaves her after a passionate night and dances with other *gopika*s (cowherdesses). She vehemently demands Krishna's complete attention and loyalty, and she envies the attention that Krishna seems to bestow upon other women. She pines for him when they are apart, longs for their union, and quarrels jealously with him when she imagines another's marks of amorousness on his body. Her friend convinces her that Krishna loves no other as much as he loves her, and finally, she abandons any modicum of ego or modesty and boldly goes to meet him. Their triumphant reunion is explicitly sensual, intimate, erotic, and fervent. At times, Radha is searingly fierce; at others, touchingly vulnerable. She is the quintessential *nayika*, the classic romantic-dramatic heroine who takes us through the entire gamut of big, complicated, messy, bold human emotions.

Jayadeva is a master of his craft, and he draws deeply from the wellsprings of the *rasa* theory elucidated in the Natyashastra, the classic text of the performing arts composed somewhere between 200 BCE and 200 CE. *Rasa*, literally meaning flavor or essence, refers to the flavor of the emotion (*bhava*) evoked by the artist, composer, or author in the audience or reader. There are nine main *rasa*s; *sringara* (beauty, love), *haasya* (mirth), *raudra* (fury), *kaarunya* (compassion), *bhibhitsa* (disgust), *bhayanaka* (terror, intense fear), *veera* (heroism), and *adhbhuta* (wonder). The prominent *rasa* in this text is *sringara rasa*. Jayadeva sets the mood with elaborate descriptions of nature and Radha and Krishna's physical beauty. The poem describes sensual-erotic love that is used as a metaphor for spiritual ecstasy.

The *Gita Govinda* was one of those rare works that almost immediately caught the imagination of the people, spreading far and wide from its eastern Indian roots, with commentaries in all parts of India within a few years of its composition. The earliest evidence of its transmission is a thirteenth-century temple inscription in Gujarat. The text was and continues to be enacted with music, drama, and dance. From drummers in the temples of southern Kerala to exquisite Basholi paintings in the northern-most part of India, from being a part of the repertoire of classical dances such as Bharatnatyam and Odissi to being a part of the spring celebration of Nepal, the *Gita Govinda* has infused an array of cultural traditions.

Jayadeva masterfully weaves undertones of mystical ecstasy with a full-throated, whole-bodied expression of sensuality unabashedly blurring lines between eros and spirituality, mysticism and emotionality. Radha emerges as an entity to be reckoned with. The ferality of her desire and her assertive-ness of expression are telling centerpieces of the poem, not creative embel-lishments for mere effect. Jayadeva wields the *sringara rasa* of the text to humanize Krishna. *Gita Govinda* is a Vaishnavite text through and through: Krishna's deific qualities are emphasized perhaps in their contrast to his human ones.

Jayadeva is an avid devotee who extols the many virtues of Krishna as Jagannatha or Lord of the World, "who takes the cosmic form at will," "who washes evil from the world in a flood of warriors' blood," and "who, moved by deep compassion, you condemn the Vedic way that ordains animal slaughter in rites of sacrifice."[10] Krishna of the *Gita Govinda* is decidedly dif-ferent from his portrayal in the Bhagavat Purana or the Bhagavad Gita. Jaya-deva's Krishna is tender, passionate, and a consummate lover who teases, flirts, dances, listens, sings, beseeches, and pines for love. Though he is all-powerful, he is also human and heroic, and his lovers embrace him as a man, not as a deity. He is also vulnerable and emotional, and he is melancholic when Radha leaves him when she is angry:

> *Her joyful responses to my touch,*
> *Trembling liquid movements of her eyes,*
> *Fragrance from her lotus mouth,*
> *A sweet ambiguous stream of words,*
> *Nectar from her red berry lips—*
> *Even when the sensuous objects are gone,*
> *My mind holds on to her in a trance.*
> *How does the wound of her desertion deepen (thus)?[11]*

By the fifteenth century, the performance of *Gita Govinda* by *devadasi*s (literal meaning: servants of god) was integrated into the temple in Puri as an integral component of worship. *Devadasi*s were accomplished artistes who dedicated their entire lives in devotional service of the deity of the temple and were ceremonially initiated as brides of the god or goddess, surrendering (or being made to surrender) their rights to marriage. They went through rigorous training in the arts and expanded the repertoire of the performing arts—especially dance forms like Bharatnatyam, Odissi, Kuchipudi, and Kathak—in vivid ways. There was a dark side to the practice as well. Families sometimes offered prepubescent girls up as *devadasi*s for many reasons, including appeasement of the village deity. The practice can be traced back to the seventh century, when the *devadasi*s came from marginalized caste communities and became consorts and courtesans of the royalty or the privileged gentry. However, this patronage came with caveats: *Devadasi*s were not accorded status as spouses, and their progeny had no legal claim to property. While some of them had a certain prestige due to their association with the temple and were able to accumulate financial resources, most *devadasi*s were exploited and subjugated for centuries. Since British colonization, many laws have been passed to abolish this practice, yet it continues in some parts of the country.

In the sixteenth century, the eminent Vaishnava mystic Chaitanya Mahaprabhu, a Brahmin saint, settled in the temple town of Puri, where he witnessed a dramatic reenactment of *Gita Govinda*. Intensely moved by the composition, he canonized the text in the Sahajya cult, deeming the erotic and sensual interplay between Radha and Krishna as allegories of spiritual ecstasy. According to Chaitanya's teachings, which integrated the philosophies of *dvaita* (dualism), *advaita* (nondualism), and *vishishta-*dvaita (qualified nondualism), all living beings, including animals and trees, are ultimately *jivatma*s (individual consciousnesses), and Krishna is the ultimate, perennial consciousness (Param-atma). Thus, the *gopika*s are *jivatma*s who long for union with the Param-atma. He emphasized bhakti as an end in itself in which devotional chanting of Krishna's name with consistency would liberate a devotee from the cycles of life and death, in which Radha-rani (Queen/Goddess Radha) was an inextricable part of "Krishna" consciousness. His teachings influenced the International Society for Krishna Consciousness (ISKCON, colloquially known as the Hare Krishna organization).

Radha-Krishna thus became inextricably intertwined in the collective imagination as part of a continuum: creation and creator, matter and spirit, transcendent and immanent, each flowing, becoming, and being the other. This esoteric spiritual fluidity was represented and celebrated in evocative ways, such as eighteenth-century Kangra- or Garhwal-style paintings depicting Krishna and Radha wearing each other's clothes, and temple festivals in which the idols of the deities are worshiped in this gender-bending, cross-dressing way. Stories were woven and narrated to highlight the oneness of Radha and Krishna. One of the stories was about how Krishna's wives wanted to test Radha's love for Krishna, so the wife gave her a glass of scalding hot milk to drink, saying it was given to her by Krishna. Radha drank it unflinching, unhurt; however, Krishna suffered burns in his throat, much to his wives' consternation,[12] proving that Radha and Krishna are both ultimately One.

Radha crossed religious boundaries, firing up the imaginations of a few Muslim rulers who commissioned artists to paint the eternal passion and the beauty of the *sringara rasa* of Krishna and Radha. Bhakti poets of all backgrounds, castes, and religions composed paeans to their love. Kazi Nazrul Islam, a Muslim imam's son from West Bengal (now Bangladesh), penned this poem in which he empathizes with Radha, admonishing Krishna for not listening to soulful entreaties of the women of Braj.

> *How devoid of compassion is the music of your flute*
> *How cruel is your failure to understand the women of Braj!*
> *Like the tears you have reduced me to*
> *Could I but make you weep too!*
> *Only then would you realize*
> *The endless heartburn born of a guru's neglect.*[13]

The long history of the development of Radha is a great example of how non-Vedic figures became integrated and appropriated into the Brahmanical pantheon. Like Radha, Krishna is not a deity in the Vedas, and is first mentioned in the seventh-century BCE Chandogya Upanishad as Krishnaya-devakiputraya (Krishna, the son of Devaki). Krishna is one of the most beloved deities, and his childhood mischief and boyhood tales in Vrindavan are a part of lore. Few figures seem to evoke the same collective emotionality he does. He is beloved as *balakrishna*, a precocious child who stole butter from neighboring homes and yet saved the village from torrential rains by lifting the mighty Govardhan Mountain with his little finger.

Like Radha, Krishna is poised on the precipices of divinity and humanity. He is relatable; when a young child, he lies to his mother when she catches him stealing; he flirts with the *gopikas*; he is loyal to his childhood friend, Sudama. At the culmination of their education in the *gurukul*, Krishna and Sudama promise to never forget each other when they have to go their separate ways. Years pass, and then Sudama's wife tells him to go meet his famous friend, as he always talks so fondly of their times together. Sudama is hesitant because now Krishna is the powerful chieftain of his clan, and Sudama is a poor farmer; would Krishna even remember their innocent childhood days? When Sudama eventually goes to meet him, having walked in the heat and dust, Krishna welcomes him with great love and affection and offers him refreshment. He playfully asks Sudama what he got him as a gift. Sudama shyly offers him a little pouch of beaten rice, *poha*, and says he remembered that it was Krishna's favorite, but he didn't offer it at first because it was too modest a gift for a mighty chieftain. Krishna takes it and eats with great gusto, and he gently chides Sudama, saying anything that is offered with love is the best gift of all. There are many stories like these, peppered with morals and ethics, that line many a child's bookshelf in India, making Krishna one of the most endearing and enduring figures.

Delving into the history of the figure of Krishna is fraught with emotionality because it involves looking into the multidimensionality of a hero and a deity. He is the *ishta-devata*, cherished deity, of millions, and has been so for millennia. He is beloved to me too, the one whom I turn to and have quiet conversations with (which is how I pray). I share this again for transparency of my own internal path into practicing holding multiplicities.

Most scholars, including nineteenth-century monk and philosopher Swami Vivekananda, expressed doubt that there was one single historical person who could be identified as Krishna. "There seem to be several Krishnas: one was mentioned in the Upanishads, another was king, another a general. All have been lumped into one Krishna. It does not matter much. The fact is, some individual comes who is unique in spirituality. Then all sorts of legends are invented around him."[14] Vivekananda also espoused the teachings of the Bhagavad Gita as being influential in his own life, so he is an example of holding both—bhakti and discernment.

The historical antecedents of Krishna form a composite of many deities that came together over centuries. Krishna's origins are from non-Vedic and non-Brahmanical backgrounds. The most prominent association is Vasudeva, a deity-hero from the Vrishni tribe. Vasudeva coalesced with the figure of Krishna, who was a popular pastoral hero of the Yadava clan. There is an image of Vasudeva on a silver coin of Agotheles the Greek in the early first century CE.[15] The emergence of Vaishnavism as an important Hindu denomination, with Vishnu as the manifestation of Brahman, happened outside the Vedic canon over centuries. In second-century CE sculptures in Bihar, he is depicted along with his brother, Balarama. Until then, Vishnu was a minor deity of the Vedas, less important than Indra or Agni. In the third-century Harivamsa, a comprehensive text on the cosmological and historical origins of Hari (another name for Krishna), Krishna is extolled as one of the ten avatars of Vishnu. This text is considered as a supplement to the Mahabharata, and scholars believe that it started as an oral tradition paying homage to the valiant feats of the pastoral heroes and was later transcribed by Vyasa.

Vaishnavism, the worship of Vishnu, became synonymous with the worship of the avatars of Vishnu, especially Rama and Krishna. This tradition was regarded as a more egalitarian, heart-centered antidote to Brahmanism, and more approachable than stringent and esoteric Shaivism. Vaishnavism was more elastic, as it integrated, absorbed, and appropriated regional, tribal deities such as Vithoba from Maharashtra and Jagannatha from Orissa. This strengthened its popular appeal across the country. Vaishnava texts were composed in Sanskrit, such as Bhagavat Purana, along with vernacular languages by the bhakti practitioners of all backgrounds, castes, and lived experiences. For instance, in the mid-seventeenth century the courtesan, scholar, and poet Muddupalani wrote *Radhika Santwanam*, an erotic epic that consists of 584 poems. This tale of Radha's longing depicts her as Krishna's aunt, an older woman in her prime and a foster parent to a woman named Ila Devi. In this tale, Radha gets Ila Devi married to Krishna even though she herself is desperately in love with him. The poems are Radha's counsel to the young bride on the intricacies of lovemaking, and a beseeching of Krishna to be a tender lover. Muddupalani describes Radha's pain and loneliness in a poignant unfolding of emotions: love, desperation, desire, and pique at Krishna for abandoning her. The poem's title is inspired by Krishna's assurance of his love for her.

Radha brought an emotionality to the legends of Krishna, humanizing a warrior-chieftain figure. The rise of Radha coincides with the period when Vaishnavism was ignited by the Bhakti uprisings all over the country. She was human enough to empathize with, boldly herself, an aspiration, and as a paramour to the divine, sacred enough to be worshiped. In contrast to the other consort in the Vaishnava tradition, Sita, Radha's stories evoked erotic pleasure as well as passionate devotion. She represented an intersection of Tantric, Shakta, and Vaishnava traditions. She was the ultimate beloved *rasika* (the heroine immersed in *sringara rasa*), unafraid to express herself in every way. In the twelfth part of the *Gita Govinda*, she invites Krishna to:

Paint a leaf on my breasts!
Put color on my cheeks!
Lay a girdle on my hips!
Twine my heavy braid with flowers!
Fix rows of bangles on my hands

And jeweled anklets on my feet!
Her yellow robed lover
Did what Radha said.[16]

The Rise and Rise of Bhakti

Bhakti *marga*, the path of devotion, has always been an integral and accessible spiritual practice for multitudes. In ancient South Asia, reverence for the goddess dates from before the Vedic period. A large number of mother goddess images and the bronze statue of a nude dancing girl from the Harappan civilization could be read as a continued veneration of "the life giving power of women and women's special relationship to reproduction, and an acceptance of their sexuality."[17] While the Brahmins used ritual to summon the Vedic gods, the village deities (*grama devatas*) were the beloved and fierce guardians of the farmers, laborers, and artisans. Bhakti, loving devotion to a personal deity, flourished after the Vedic period. The divine was imagined, experienced, and worshiped with heart-centered, full-throated expressiveness, a way of accessing the divine that became integrated as one of the three yogic paths espoused by Krishna in the Bhagavad Gita. This was one of the ways that yoga and "religion" overlapped, via deity worship in the practice of bhakti *marga*. Thus the austere sramanic contemplative asceticism that was synonymous with yoga slowly expanded to include the orthodoxy of Brahmanism as well as the heterodoxy of those who challenged the hierarchies of caste, class, and gender.

Bhakti yoga exuberantly opened doors to the sacred and the exalted. There was no priest, no meddling middle person needed to create and express outpourings of love to the personal deity or the *ishta-devata*. There was no need for ostentatious displays of wealth or elaborate performance of ritual. There was no necessity for scholarly and analytical dissections of the texts. Anyone could practice anywhere and anyhow. While caste posed obstacles to access to Sanskrit texts or temples, devotees intent and rooted in a personal, visceral connection with the divine persisted and tore down barriers of gender, class, and caste. The maid, the courtesan, the wife, the weaver, the potter, the blind, even the wicked rose up in passionate, explicit, heartfelt, and fierce longing for union with the Cherished One. They were sometimes feral in their tone of expression. Unlike the stringent austerities of ascetics, the body was very much a part of the connection, the vessel of deliverance and the medium of expression. The mundaneness of existence, of everyday life, was transformed with prayer, conversation, song, and dance. Form and name, matter and spirit, earth and heaven danced together in a delicious, ferocious, delirious way in Bhakti poetry.

Ego was cast aside, shame was broken down, tearing down the walls between the sacred and the mundane. Everybody was called in to witness, to participate, and to experience love and surrender. The root verb of bhakti is *bhaj*, which means to have recourse to or partake in. The divine was a lover, a friend, a spouse, a partner; the relationship between the god-goddess and the devotee was intimate and urgent. There are nine forms of bhakti: *kirtana* (hymns); *sravana* (listening to the names of the divine), *smarana* (remembering), *pada-smarana* (being at the feet of the deity, both metaphorically and literally), *vandana* (prayer), *archana* (worship through offerings), *dasya* or *seva* (can be translated as service), *sakhya* (friendship), and Atma-nivedana (complete surrender). Bhakti poetry often expressed the emotion of *viraha*, the yearning for union and the utter anguish of separation from the *ishta-devata*. Radha was one of the sublime creations of this aspect of the Bhakti period.

Bhakti was not sentimentality devoid of *jnana* or karma. Bhakti embraced knowledge for what it offered, a certain insight into transcendence, and yet was not tied to it; bhakti wasn't contained by books and scripture and pontification. While some broke away from societal norms and socially sanctioned relationships of marriage and family, others worked within these parameters. For some the eros, the mundane, and the spiritual were not separate; one led to the other, one merged with the other. Radha the icon was borne from this heady concoction of bhakti, an alchemy of the human craving for something transcendent while reveling in the *rasa*, the richly textured, juicy emotionality devoid of ego and guilt. Like most ancient figures, she is a composite of many heroines, both historical and mythical. As the patriarchal, gender-normative orthodoxy of Brahmanism spread and gained momentum during the Puranic period (from around 500 CE onward), the dominant portrayal of Radha transformed into the subdued consort-goddess of Krishna that overshadowed the far more sensual, colorful, humane narrative.

Bhakti was expansive and could be practiced toward the formless (without manifest attributes) *nirguna* Brahman, or toward the *saguna* Brahman (one with form and shape), depending on the practitioner's inclination and imagination. The *saguna* bhakti could be directed toward a particular deity. Different traditions were based on which deity was at the center of religious life. Those who worshipped Vishnu and his incarnations like Rama and Krishna were Vaishnavas, those oriented toward Shiva were Shaivas, and those who worshipped the Goddess and her manifestations were Shaktas. While the *saguna* bhakti saints reveled in a personal, almost intimate relationship with their *ishta-devata*, in the *nirguna* bhakti of Kabir and the Sikh Guru Nanak, the quest for eternal divinity was not limited by form or image and was unfettered by religion or region.

Kabir, a Muslim weaver who was perhaps the most beloved *nirguna* bhakti saint, decried the limitations and hierarchies of the caste system, the corruption of priests and mullahs, and the impositions of both Brahmanism and Islam. His conceptualization of *jivanmrit*, literally meaning being dead while alive,[18] was a reminder that moksha was not something one aspired to after death, but an aspirational ideal for the way one lived, with rationality, meaning, and purpose. He composed couplets or *dohas* that emphasized simplicity of practice, doing away with dogmatism, pomp, and circumstance. His poetry was rife with metaphors inspired by his craft as a weaver and exhibited an extraordinary example of his prowess and insight as a yogi. In one *doha*, he compares the warp and weave of the blanket to the five elements (*tattvas*)—fire, water, earth, air, and ether; and the three *gunas* (*sattva, rajas,* and *tamas*). He then goes on to assert his *jatan* (intentional effort) in the way he has weaved the tapestry, a metaphor for how he has lived his life with a strong ethical core, even more than the so-called pious and wise men.

The eight petaled lotus is the spinning wheel
With five tattvas *and three* gunas, *He makes the blanket*[19]

The different Bhakti factions were often antagonistic toward one another. The Vaishnavite clashed with the Shakta, who criticized the Shaivite, who returned the sentiments with equal fervor, with each claiming their beloved deity to be superior and thus a more authentic embodiment of the divine. There is an overidealization of a pre-Islamic India as a peaceful, utopian haven for diverse spiritual pursuits. However, there are many textual and archaeological sources that point to the violence among the different faith traditions prior to the Islamic rulers. For instance, the twelfth-century Kashmiri text *Rajatarangini* mentions one of Ashoka's sons, Jalauka, a Shaivite (unlike his Buddhist father), who destroyed Buddhist monasteries. The Divyadana (around the second century CE), a Buddhist Sanskrit text, reports the prosecution of sramanas by the Brahmin ruler Pushyamitra Sungha, who marched out with a large army destroying stupas and monasteries and announced a prize of one hundred dinars for the head of every sramana.[20]

Bhakti can be liberatory, lending spiritual and emotional agency. It can also maintain caste hierarchies. Many of the Brahmanical traditions, temples, and spaces were and are not welcoming of people from all caste identities. Temples were built to display, experience, and practice bhakti. They were also statements of political power and prosperity, a testament to the ruler's wealth, artistic sensibilities, and sophistication. Many were showcases of artisanship and grandeur patronized by wealthy landowners, merchants, or the royal family. The temple was a monument that in many ways maintained the caste system. While it was the center of communal gatherings for the caste-privileged, the Dalits, the Shudras, and other caste-oppressed communities were (and still are) not allowed entry into temples with Puranic deities and/or Brahmin priests. Even though they provided the labor for the transport of material and construction, many temples prevented them from entering the inner areas where the deity was established. There also have been ardent devotees like Kanaka in the fifteenth century, who was denied entry by priests into the famed Krishna temple in Udupi, Karnataka, because of his caste status. Legend has it that his bhakti-infused poetry moved Krishna so deeply that his *moorthi* (idol) turned to face the west so that Kanaka could see his beloved deity without any obstacles. Even to this day, the idol faces west, unlike other temples where the idols face east.

The Dalits, Shudras, and other caste-marginalized communities had (and continue to have) their own temples, deities, and modes of worship. During times of war, when a king invaded a rival's territory, the temple was the first monument that was either looted, destroyed completely, or refurbished so as to establish the king's own deity or tradition as the ruling deity of the land. For instance, the famous Thanjavur temple in modern Tamil Nadu was built by Rajaraja of the Chola dynasty after the invasion of their rivals, the Cheras and Pandyas.

Regardless of the political maneuverings or perhaps because of it, bhakti as a practice was here to stay. There are many theories for the spontaneous Bhakti movement uprisings; it may have been a response to the growing political power as well as the monotheistic and relatively egalitarian ideas of the Muslim invaders, and/or the increasing rigidity of the caste system. It could also have been due to the emerging affluence of artisans and traders, which spurred their aspirations to have the status and privileges of the Brahmins and the Kshatriyas. The reasons for the movement may be many, but Bhakti irrevocably revolutionized the cultural, social, and spiritual landscape of multitudes.

Some of the most prominent Bhakti saints are folks from all castes and classes, such as Mirabai, a Rajput royal princess, and Janabai, a Shudra poetess in the thirteenth century. Since women's labor was always an integral part of home-based artisan production, there was a bhakti emphasis on the life of the householder and their domestic responsibilities.[21] There are many poems that describe a woman's drudgery, which often stood in the way of spiritual and intellectual emancipation and the much-anticipated liberation, when one finally broke free of all obstacles. Janabai, one of the most beloved poets of the Varkari sects of Maharashtra, worked in the home of a householder named Namdev. She wove her household responsibilities into her poetry, sometimes with tongue in cheek, beseeching her beloved deity Vithoba to grant her freedom:

> *O God, my darling*
> *Do me a favor and kill my mother-in-law*
> *I will feel lonely when she is gone*
> *But you will be a good god won't you*
> *And kill my father-in-law*
> *I will be glad when he is gone*
> *But you will be a good god won't you*
> *And kill my sister-in-law*
> *I will be free when she is gone*
> *I will pick up my begging bowl*
> *And be on my way*
> *Let them drop dead says Jani*
> *Then we will be left alone*
> *Just you and me.*[22]

Although there was a passionate and concerted rejection of hierarchies, caste and gender continued to influence the lives and works of Bhakti poet-saints. Many of the caste-privileged Bhakti poets (men) exhibit a vivid awareness of their own positionality and passionately decried caste and gender hierarchies. They viewed caste and their own gender as obstacles that harm all of humanity and sought a just and equal society devoid of caste distinctions. There was a concerted and intentional struggle "in all sorts of ways to shed pomp and privilege. The women broke every rule of Manu's codebook for good wives, almost as if they had the book open in front of them, turning the palm leaves and ticking them off."[23] Some of them defied rules, ate with avarna folks, and saw the divine in every being regardless of caste. The sixteenth-century Bhakti poet Eknath was a Brahmin who challenged the elite in many ways, acknowledging all human beings from all castes as being equal in the presence of the divine.

Women and caste-oppressed folks, on the other hand, had to confront multiple patriarchal norms. Folks like Andal rejected the shackles of domesticity completely, viewing them as burdensome obstacles in their paths. Others, like Janabai and Mirabai, were coerced into marriage and had to repeatedly push back against patriarchal gender norms and societal taunts when they rebelled and refused to conform. Janabai's dark, humorous plea to her beloved deity Vithoba reveals the frustration incited by all the demands she might have had on her time and life, demands that kept her from doing what she was drawn to the most: bhakti.

The body was a vehicle of transcendence, fluid and transient, ever-changing and thus superficial in the quest for the eternality of the sacred and sublime. In the next two chapters, Akka Mahadevi's startling life choices in the thirteenth century and Piro in the eighteenth century will reveal their divergent perspectives on how they viewed the physical body in the quest for union with their beloved. Thus bhakti was the path of heterodoxy, dissent, revolt, radical and passionate love and devotion for the supraordinary by ordinary and extraordinary people.

The interconnectedness and intersections of spiritual, economic, and political systems cannot be denied or ignored. The Bhakti movement was also not devoid of the impact of misogyny, of the imposition of political power, of caste supremacy or imperialism. Class and caste continued to play a central role in who got access to which deity and how. While Kabir's poems decried the shackles of caste and class, they do reveal a mistrust of women as impediments to a man's enlightenment. In a few verses he says "woman destroys three merits when she comes near a man; devotion, salvation and divine knowledge," so she is thus "a pit of hell."[24] Tulsidas, the sixteenth-century Brahmin Bhakti poet, composed *Ramcharitmanas* (the story of Rama) in Awadhi, a language far more accessible than Sanskrit; but the text highlighted the legitimacy of the caste system. In this composition, in *Aranyakanda* (book 3), Rama describes Brahmins as deserving of reverence even when they lack virtue and character; Shudras, on the other hand, do not deserve respect even when they are learned and virtuous.[25]

People in power from every faith and religion have always tried to weaponize anything that can be used to maintain the status quo. While bhakti broke down a few barriers, corruption and greed for power creeped through the crevices and resurrected in different ways. Wars have been fought, and even today, we witness the world burning for different names of the divine. Politics and religion are increasingly intertwined in India and the diaspora, where the staunch supporters of Modi are even called *bhakt*s or devotees. It is imperative to practice discernment while practicing bhakti and to ensure critical insight into how one can be corralled by faith traditions.

Key Takeaways

Rasa as Resistance

Radha's stories illuminate a quintessential human longing: to belong to another, be it a connection to the sacred or to another human being. The poets, the singers, the dancers, the artists, the bhakti practitioners connect to her as an eternal icon of that innate yearning. She is neither fully human nor completely a deity. She is not bogged down by the householder tradition, nor is she pursuing the ascetic ideal. In all the stories, she is a lover, a woman with agency. She has real, human emotions; she is greedy for her lover's attention and touch. She enthralls and is enthralled by Krishna, the hero-deity, but she does not worship him as one. She is his equal. She is considered as a goddess only in the later Puranic texts. While many yoga practitioners may know of the Bhagavad Gita, texts like the *Gita Govinda* are lesser known. Both feature Krishna; one is situated in the epic Mahabharata, and the other is from a poet-saint, Jayadeva. The boundaries between eros and spirituality were less rigid than they are today. One's body was a vehicle for pleasure, for *sringara rasa*, as well as an expression of worship of the divine.

The divine and the human were both separate and united. Bhakti was an expression of love and longing in all its forms, moving people across religious, gender, and even caste boundaries. Kabir, a Muslim weaver, was very moved by Vaishnavism and considered Rama not as an idol to be worshiped in a temple but someone whom he could address directly as a symbol of the divine. Dominant cultures demand categorization. Capitalism assigns value to how one can be efficient. We are conditioned to compartmentalize or simplify our complexities of who we are as humans. Our work in the world, our identities, our emotional lives, our thoughts and opinions, our relationships with each other, our spiritual aspirations are defined as disparate rather than fluid, flowing into and nourishing each other. Therefore, an ongoing exploration of liminality in ourselves and the other can offer rich insights, bridging our notions of who we are as humans and expanding the definitions of the sacred as veritable extensions of that experience.

Brahmanism, Appropriation, and Sanitization

Radha was first mentioned as a bucolic folk heroine, someone whom Krishna was exceptionally fond of. The later Sanskrit Puranas transformed her into an incarnation of Lakshmi, and then she was Radha-rani, the goddess-queen of the Vaishnavas. A fiercely independent tribal heroine thus became a tamer version, a consort of a male deity, which neutralized a subversive narrative of sexual and spiritual agency. Radha has a very different flavor from Durga or Kaali. Even though the mythical roots of Radha and Krishna are based outside Vedic tradition, the appropriation of both into a larger pantheon is how Brahmanism spread rapidly. Jagannatha in Odisha and Vithoba in Maharashtra started as local deities. As they gained popularity, their status was elevated by the claim that they are forms of a pan-Indian Krishna. This process of linking a local deity with a transregional one is a strategy to subsume the individual tribal identity under the unified whole, absorbing entire mythologies and cultural traditions into a pan-Indian one with its embedded hierarchies of caste and gender. Thus tribal traditions and stories were absorbed by what later came to be known as the Hindu religion.

Radha became another form of a Hindu *devi*. Her sensual relationship with Krishna was interpreted as an allegory, the yearning of *jivatma* to unite with the Param-atma. While this analogy may be useful in making the metaphysical abstraction of consciousness more accessible, there is also a dire need to uplift sheer enjoyment, *rasa*, especially today when patriarchal systems and institutions censor expression of femme and gender-expansive folks and women's sexualities. Embracing pleasure for the sake of pleasure is shrouded in shame and guilt, even today. What would shift in our understanding of emancipation if we centered the full-blooded sensuality, the *sringara rasa* that Radha represents?

Bhakti and Viveka (Discernment): Holding Multiplicities

Bhakti disrupts hierarchies, rejecting the notion that one would need a priest, a scholar, or any middle person between the *bhakt* (practitioner) and the divine. It is a heart-centered connection of the mundane to the sacred, the individual to the collective through the depth and resonance of *bhava* (emotions). There is simply no stringent requirement or ritual, nor are there specific rules for how one can express loving devotion. The practices of bhakti are manifold, rooted in culture, faith, and religion. It is not to be confused with the sappy sacchariness of sentimentality; it is an honest, heartfelt, authentic, relationship-building practice with *saguna* or *nirguna* Brahman.

Bhakti softens austerities for householders and offers solace, belonging, and an anchor during turbulent times. However, we need to acknowledge its contradictions and paradoxes, too. People can also be corralled by faith traditions, and one has to practice discernment while practicing bhakti. Emotionality can coexist with *viveka*, discernment; in fact it is imperative, or we run into the very real danger of idolatry. Wars have been fought—and are being fought—over religion and faith, and extremism is on the rise. As yoga practitioners, more than ever there is an impetus to hold the tension between bhakti and unquestioning dogma-ridden faith, especially now when religious and/or spiritual narratives are co-opted and weaponized to impose dominance and cultural hegemony.

Bhakti can be liberatory, lending spiritual and emotional agency. It can also maintain caste hierarchies. Many of the Brahmanical traditions, temples, and spaces have not welcomed people from all caste identities. Hindutva is no longer a fringe ideal to be scoffed at by the intelligentsia; it has been institutionalized and globalized in its influence and presence. In the context of bhakti yoga, there is an undermining of the influence of other faiths and religions in yoga, highlighting Brahmanical orthodoxy, such as an emphasis on Sanskrit without acknowledgement of its complex and oppressive caste history. By studying the origins of texts from multiple sources and engaging in critical discourse, we can unravel the history of power dynamics and how they persist or manifest in contemporary systems and institutions. By doing so, we learn how narratives are shaped and sustained through centuries. If one studies the histories of mythical figures and interrogates the evolution of myths, oral and written, one learns about the multihued perspectives and worldviews of the storytellers. Reflecting on our own culturally conditioned *samskaras* regarding the complex truths of our faith or religious practices is a critical and yet underemphasized part of yoga studies.

Bhakti itself cannot be painted with one broad brushstroke, as practitioners have experienced and practiced it in such different ways through centuries. There have been sharp divergences between people of a particular bhakti sect and between different faith traditions. As a yoga community, we need to counter the deliberate obfuscation of the complexity of history, separate religion and state, distinguish liberatory truths from oppressive ideology, and study the story of a story as it traverses time and space.

Summary

Radha is a representation of bhakti, the practice of loving devotion. Her earliest story as a tribal heroine is absorbed into Vaishnava Puranic literature as a consort-goddess. This shines a light onto the dynamism between the folk/tribal tradition and the pan-Hindu tradition. Even though bhakti rebels against orthodox rituals, it still gets co-opted by dominant culture and castes. Hence, it is imperative to practice holding multiplicities and cultivating discernment into how bhakti is deployed to maintain hegemony.

These are the questions we need to ask ourselves and others if we are to reclaim and recenter the open-hearted embrace of bhakti:

- If bhakti (or devotion in other religions) is such a healing balm, why is the world today sharply divided and polarized along faith and religious traditions?

- How is faith hijacked to establish power and hegemony?

- Can one's bhakti flourish at the expense of another? Where does faith end and oppression begin?

- How can contemporary bhakti yoga practitioners learn from the historical examples provided to challenge contemporary social oppression?

- Why does misuse or abuse of power persist in communities ostensibly committed to egalitarianism?

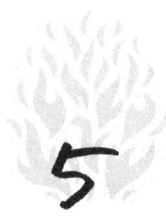

5

THE NAKED TRUTH TELLERS

This was the end, or was it the beginning? She knew it was time to be united with her Chennamallikarjuna, her Lord of the Hill, her Beloved, fragrant as the white jasmine, her Shiva. Fire in her eyes, ice in her voice, she turned to Kaushika, the one whom they had forced her to marry when she was a child. You have failed me for the last time. Three times, I have forgiven your transgressions. You promised me that I will not be disturbed in my prayer, in my sadhana, *that I will not be kept away from meeting my guru and the wandering mendicants, and that I shall be free and unhindered to live the way I like. You have broken all three promises, Kaushika. You have come in the way of my prayer, you have prevented me from meeting with my guru, and you have questioned the way I live. You have gone back on the conditions I set to marry you. Our marriage is thus void and null. I am leaving you to join my true husband of my heart, Shiva, please step aside.*

Kaushika, her husband, the chieftain, fell silent. She started shedding everything. There was precision and grace in her actions. She removed her jewelry, her bangles, and her anklet, one by one, without a grimace, a cool flame seemed to light her from within. She shed her clothes, every piece of it without any hesitation, every action intentional and deliberate in the effort to be finally without any barriers, without anything that could come in between her and the Creator. She unbraided her long, dark tresses, letting them loose, free and wild. She began walking out. The maids called out, Akka, sister, what are you doing? Where will you go? She paid no heed and kept on walking. The people came out to watch, some bowed their heads and folded their hands in a namaste, some looked away in respect, while others pointed and jeered at her, a naked woman walking the streets in broad daylight. She has lost her mind, they said. She has no shame, they said. Some hurled stones, while others wounded with words. Some hushed the others, silencing the abuses hurled her way. They knew she was a Shiva devotee and was married to their chieftain. She was resolute, none of them mattered, none of their words or actions changed her pace. She kept walking, head held high, her gait unhurried and unchanged. She went to her parents' home to bid them goodbye.

Her mother, aghast at her wanton disregard for modesty, implored her, you will be reviled as a charlatan, they will call you a madwoman, a bad woman, please wear some clothes. Her father, a Shiva devotee like her, appealed to her, you can stay with us and do your poojas without any disturbance, please do not go out into the wild. She listened politely and did not respond. Her mind was made up, she touched their feet with great respect, thanked them for their concern, and turned around and left in search of her Shiva. She was free at last, a seeker and a lover, a devotee and a bride of Chennamallikarjuna, the Lord as Fragrant as the White Jasmine. She would be clad henceforth only in her quest to be united with Shiva. This was her beginning. She was Akka Mahadevi.

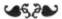

Naked unto the Light

Akka Mahadevi was born to Nirmala Shetty and Sumati around 1130 CE in the Shivamogga district of Karnataka, one of the southern states of India. Her parents were avid devotees of Shiva. She may have had a life-altering mystical experience when she was a young girl and had a guru who guided her in spiritual pursuits in her early years. Mahadevi grew up worshiping the *lingam*, the symbol of Shiva, and considered herself to be betrothed to him. This sort of voluntary "bridal mysticism,"[1] in which the devotee considers the deity as a spouse or lover, was a part of Bhakti culture and occurred across all genders.

From Andal to Kabir, Bhakti poets often referred to their *ishta-devata* as a beloved. This was different from the *devadasis* whose families offered them to the temple or who were born into a family of *devadasi*s. Bridal mysticism was passionate devotion from a woman or femme's own volition; no one forced the devotee to accept the divine as her spouse. Instead there was a deep, intrinsic longing to be in connection and union with one's *ishta-devata*. This yearning sometimes took on an intense intimacy, a fervent imagination, and, dare we say, an experience of a personal relationship with the divine. In Mahadevi's mind and heart, she was already wedded to her Chennamallikarjuna, the Lord of the Peaks, Shiva; so for her, to marry a mortal was a tremendous hindrance. She might never have married if she was not coerced into it by Kaushika, a Jain chieftain who saw her one day and was besotted with her form and grace.

Kaushika tried everything—from confessing his ardent love, to bribery, to blackmail—to convince Mahadevi to marry him. She relented when she heard her beloved parents' plea to save their lives from the wrath of a scorned Kaushika. She put forth three conditions for her marriage: She would not be deterred in any way from her *sadhana* and *pooja*, she would not be prevented from meeting her gurus, and he would never get in the way of how she lived her life. Kaushika agreed to all three conditions, and for some time, all was well. He promised her she could pursue her path of bhakti, meet with the visiting mendicants, and live as she pleased. However, Kaushika, filled with entitlement as a patriarch, broke his promises one by one. Mahadevi forgave him twice, but after the third time he broke his promise, she finally held him to her premarriage conditions, tore down all the barriers of relationships, of societal expectations, of gender norms, and left him to go seek the ultimate union with her beloved, Shiva.

I am in love with the One
Who knows no death, no evil, no form
Who knows no place, no space.
No beginning, no end.
Who knows no fears nor the snares
Of this world.
I am in love with my husband,
My Lord, Chennamallikarjuna.[2]

Mahadevi knew where she wanted to commence her pilgrimage, her solitary quest for *aikya*, union with Shiva. She had heard about Kalyana, the town where the illustrious, radical Shaivite teachers Basavanna and Allama Prabhu lived with other Shiva *sharanas*, the ones who sought refuge in the worship of Shiva. She had heard that this sect—also known as the Veerashaivas, the brave Shiva devotees—were a revolutionary group who rejected the centrality of the Vedas, the crushing constraints of varna-ashrama-dharma, and the alleged spiritual superiority of the Brahmins. She had heard that all devotees were welcome without any differentiation and were accorded equal access to philosophical discourse, debates, and discussion. Basavanna's radical advocacy for intercaste marriage and widow remarriage had spread far and wide. Most importantly, she yearned for community, to be with like-hearted people with their shared bhakti and zeal for *aikya*, union with their beloved Shiva.

Mahadevi walked more than five hundred miles through villages and thick forests, braving the brutal vagaries of the elements. How did people react to this sight of a naked, unabashed young woman, her disheveled long hair almost sweeping the ground, walking with a fierce steadfastness? Not much is known of how she accomplished this feat or about her experiences and encounters along the way. Did people greet her with respect or jeer at her nude form? Did they offer her water and food or shun her as an ill omen? Did they leave her alone, or were some inspired to follow her? We will never know the details of her arduous journey, but she did eventually reach Kalyana.

In Kalyana, word had reached Basavanna and Allama Prabhu, the two principal leaders of the Shiva *sharanas* (an informal name given to the devotees of Shiva), that Mahadevi was on her way to meet them. Legend has it that when she entered the room called the Anubhava Mantapa, Hallowed Hall of Experience, everyone fell silent. While Basavanna smiled at her with a welcoming warmth, Allama Prabhu was skeptical and began asking her questions, challenging her in front of all the sect members. Whether he did so to establish her credibility for the rest of the group or to ensure her intention for himself, the questioning itself was long. In the fifteenth-century text

Sunya Sampadne (Attainment of the Void), there is a summary of the initial exchange between Allama Prabhu and Mahadevi. When he asked her why she was there in Kalyana, Mahadevi replied that she was there as a daughter-in-law of the house, hinting at her right to be there, a place where other Shiva devotees resided. When asked why she had left her mortal husband, she eloquently stated:

What use have I of husbands who die and decay
Throw them into the kitchen fires.
My Lord Chennamallikarjuna, He is my husband.[3]

Allama pushed her more with an age-old question. Why did she, so young and beautiful, leave her husband, Kaushika, and pursue this path? Why was she naked but at the same time covered up by her hair? Mahadevi addressed his concerns head-on, saying that she hadn't betrayed Kaushika's trust; he had broken his promises. She had only seen the face of Shiva "in every pebble and every leaf" and she was His, with her whole body and her whole heart.[4] She continued, saying her body was not her own, and a mere cloth would not cover and conceal her nakedness from the One Who Is Everywhere. The only reason she covered her body with her hair was for the world outside so that people did not mistake what they saw in her body as her real identity. When Allama heard this, he accused her of speaking of the body as if it didn't exist, which he said made her a hypocrite, "like a dead body that declares itself dead . . . like curdled milk that claims sweetness,"[5] doubting her sincerity and rectitude.

Mahadevi calmly responded that when one wakes up from a dream in which one has died and talks about it, it was like the dead who spoke of one's own death, and that when curdled milk is boiled, there is still sweetness in it, meaning that regardless of her appearance she was steadfastly dedicated in her bhakti with her body, mind, heart, and spirit. All were impressed with her eloquence and quick wit. Allama applauded her maturity, and he warmly and respectfully called her Akka, which means elder sister in Kannada, the regional language of Karnataka.

Basavanna said:

A sarane [female Shiva devotee] like Mahadevi Akka
Needs no encumbrances at all,
O, hail! Mahadevi Akka![6]

Basavanna's respectful acceptance of Mahadevi's stature as an equal, as a *sarane*, enabled Akka Mahadevi to reside in Kalyana for some time, where she met with other devotees before leaving for the next part of her journey. From there she proceeded to Srishaila, a remote temple town surrounded by forests and caves where dedicated yogis pursued their *sadhana* with great rigor. There she lived an austere ascetic's life, in quiet contemplation and prayer. When her parents and Kaushika visited, they tried to dissuade her from shutting herself away from the world in such physical hardship, but she was determined and sent them away. Here in the remote caves she finally attained what she had longed for, what she had fought for, what she had sacrificed all her mortal relationships for, what she had dreamed about, what she had spoken about in her *vachana*s (prose poems). She attained *aikya*: oneness, union with her *ishta-devata*, Lord of the Peaks, Chennamallikarjuna.

Akka Mahadevi was a prolific poet, composing nearly 355 *vachana*s that were spontaneous, heartfelt, passionate outpourings or utterances. These compositions were not *smriti* (that which is remembered), nor were they *shruthi* (that which is heard); they sprang from a different canon altogether. They did not adhere to the grammatical rules of prose, nor were they traditional poetry. *Vachana*s were what we might today call spoken-word poetry, with a fresh and fiery cadence, lucidity, and rhythm that galvanized people from all castes, creeds, classes, and genders. Akka Mahadevi, Basavanna, Allama Prabhu, and nearly three hundred other Shiva *sharana*s composed around twenty thousand *vachana*s in the twelfth century, challenging existing societal paradigms. They addressed their *ishta-devata*, Shiva, in lyrical, profound language that touched and moved people from all backgrounds, from leather tanners to farmers, from fishermen to cowherds, from laborers to potters. The beauty of the *vachana*s resonated deeply because the *vachanakars* (the composers) also practiced what they preached and defied many of the prevailing oppressive systems.

Bhakti: Beyond Body, Gender, and Caste

Around five hundred years before Mahadevi was born, there was political turbulence in the southern region of India when the Kalabhras dynasty, descendants of Tamil-speaking tribal warriors, overthrew the powerful Shaivite rule of the Cholas and the Pandyas. The Kalabhras were staunch critics of the temple-building Brahmin orthodoxy, and they welcomed Buddhists and Jains, as the two religions were considered to be more egalitarian alternatives. However, it was not easy to subvert deeply embedded Brahmanical orthodoxy. Even though the Kalabhras offered refuge and patronage to the two heterodox religions, by the fifth century Brahmanism prevailed except in the southern regions, which presented the last frontiers of resistance. Elsewhere, the norms of Brahmanism were deeply entrenched in the socioeconomic ethos of the people. While castes could theoretically be initiated into Buddhism or Jainism, prohibition of marriage between jaatis and prevention of widow remarriage persisted as forms of taboo.

During this period of religious and political upheaval, Basavanna was born to a Brahmin family. He soon grew into a precocious child who was fluent in Sanskrit and well-versed in the Vedas and other texts. He was a rebel from the very beginning who questioned the caste system. According to lore, he tore off his *janeu*—a white thread that serves as the Brahmin man's symbol of caste initiation—and left home in a quest for a guru's guidance. In his travels he had meaningful encounters with Kashmir and Nayanar Shaivism and explored Buddhist philosophy. He integrated the three traditions with a sharp critique and a departure from the tenets of Vedic Brahmanism, and he founded his own radical bhakti path called "the brave devotees of Shiva," Veerashaivas. This new syncretic doctrine rejected the centrality of the Vedas, fire rituals, the incessant temple building, and the oppression of varna-ashrama-dharma. The Veerashaiva movement burst forward with their revolutionary ideas of intercaste marriages and integration of people across castes and genders, welcoming all into their sect. One of the popular practices Basavanna introduced was the introduction of wearing the *lingam* (*ishta-linga*) on a thread or necklace. Anyone across all castes could wear one as a reminder to be steadfast in one's devotion to Shiva. Even though Basavanna was a Sanskrit scholar, he used the vernacular language, Kannada, to compose *vachana*s to render them more accessible for the multitudes, disrupting the elitism of the Brahmin scholars.

The Veerashaivas, later called the Lingayats, subverted the purity practices of the Brahmins, even refusing to eat food cooked by them as a sort of a role reversal. They gained immense popularity among the avarnas and the Shudras, especially in Karnataka (my home state in India), where they thrive to this day. After Basavanna's death, many of the more orthodox Lingayats adopted mainstream casteist traditions such as the establishment of the Panchacharas (five codes of conduct), vegetarianism, and the prohibition of alcohol consumption. This type of adoption of savarna practices by the middle tier of the jaatis was called Brahminization or Sanskritization.[7] During Basavanna's time, however, there was a definite anti-Brahmin stance that was appreciated by all those who were thwarted and repressed by the Brahmins and the Kshatriyas. Basavanna witnessed the acute shortcomings of a society that was tilted steeply in favor of the caste-privileged, and he wanted to cultivate seekers and leaders. Thus, he established the Anubhava Mantapa, a secular gathering place of devotees and scholars from every lived experience. This was why, when Akka Mahadevi decided to begin her pilgrimage, she knew she would not be turned away when she arrived there.

Basavanna staunchly opposed endogamy and arranged a marriage between two young Shiva *sharana*s, a Shudra tanner and a Brahmin's daughter. This was one of the most rebellious acts of that time, and it created many enemies for Basavanna. He pushed other boundaries, including that of gender. Many of the *vachana*s proclaim an androgynous quality, a transcendence of the social and cultural constructs of the gender binary. He taught that the shedding of all extraneous markers is a process of undergoing "divestments, as preparations for receiving god's love":[8]

Look here, dear fellow;
I wear these men's clothes
Only for you,
Sometimes I am man,
Sometimes I am woman,
O Lord Kudalasangamadeva [Shiva]
I'll make wars for you
But I'll be your devotee's bride.[9]

While it is important that we do not impose modern definitions and understandings of gender and sexuality on historical or mythical figures, it is also important for us as yoga practitioners to know about variations and heterogeneity of perspectives with regard to gender. The essences of the teachings are rooted in the perennial truth of Atma, the notion that the physical body is transient and temporary, and the precept that form and matter (prakriti) undergo change and thus do not represent the complete truth of the human experience. If Sulabha's exchange with Janaka in chapter 3 was a good example of inquiry into gender within the Upanishadic philosophy, Basavanna and his cohort represented the Bhakti context.

Many Bhakti saints considered gender and all the norms associated with it to be a sociocultural construct that could be challenged and subverted in countless ways. The way of bhakti was a way of rebellion against an artificial propriety imposed by those in power. This way was reflected in poems such as the one by Basavanna quoted above, and in the practitioners' complete disregard for societal constraints as they simply moved about in the world, like Akka Mahadevi's embrace of nakedness as a way of life.

Being naked was not a complete anomaly for practitioners, as it was an expression and practice of *vairagya* (nonattachment), an ascetic ideal. Jainism was prevalent in Karnataka during Mahadevi's lifetime. Thus she most likely had come into contact with the Digambaras, a sect of Jain monks among whom being "skyclad" or naked was an extension of renunciation; but they did not let women enter their sect or monastery. The Shvetam-bara (white-clad) sect of Jain monks, on the other hand, did accept women, but they had to be clothed. Thus, while nudity was revered and celebrated among male monks as a disregard for physical attachments, women had to be clothed and had a far more stringent set of rules to follow. Akka Mahadevi's nudity was a radical denouncement of any sort of patriarchal imposition.

Practitioners from varying social backgrounds have experienced the body in the expression of bhakti in such different ways over the centuries. Although men like Basavanna and Kabir, the former a *saguna bhakt* and the latter a *nirguna bhakt*, faced challenges and were challenged by societal norms, they were able to oppose caste and religious dogma. However, as men they had some level of privilege and comfort. Women, on the other hand, not only had to denounce their caste affiliation and familial relation-ships, they also had to tear down the metaphorical and literal veils on their bodies. Some of them quite literally shed all their clothes like Mahadevi, while others, like Mirabai, refused to participate in *sati*, a practice that was prevalent in the Rajput clan she belonged to.

Mahadevi rejected her husband's sexual advances and walked out of her marriage. For some, like Muddupalani and Piro (discussed in the next chapter), the body was a vehicle of devotional expression, of *bhava*, where the *rasa* was felt in a seamless continuum of the spiritual and the sensual. This was especially true of caste-marginalized folks who were oppressed and abused by those in power, but who within their own spaces were unfettered by the restraints of Brahminical puritanism.

Akka Mahadevi embraced the body. Her nudity was a reclamation of the ultimate expression of rebellious freedom. She walked bare, breasts and hair exposed to the sun, undeterred by the wind or the censorship of human eyes, fierce in her assuredness of who she was, a spirited devotee with only one goal: union with her beloved Shiva. No other opinion mattered. Her *vachanas* definitively described the body as an embodiment of her fiery and eloquent longing for union.

While such statements of revolt by women in the pursuit of emancipation were not typical of the time, they were not entirely anomalies either. Two centuries later and thousands of miles away, Lal Ded—a fourteenth-century mystic poet from Kashmir, beloved to Hindus as Lalleswari and to Muslims as Lal-arifa—also left her abusive husband in her quest for emancipation. Often portrayed as a wandering, naked mendicant, she was deeply inspired by Shaivism, Buddhism, Tantra, yoga, and Sufism. She composed *vakh*s, spontaneous utterances, with imagery that articulated yogic and Tantric insight into the body-mind-spirit continuum. Both Lal Ded and Mahadevi prevailed over immense personal and systemic barriers to pursue their goals, and they transformed the Bhakti landscape through their spontaneous, ingenious outpourings. Their words reverberate with a fierceness and resilience that resonate to this day.

Key Takeaways

Lean into the Power of the Spoken Word

From the *vachana*s of the Shiva *sharana*s to Lalla's *vakh*s, the beauty and the power of many oral traditions are remembered and revered in certain communities. Yet they are not very well-known in mainstream yoga or religious studies, except among a few scholars. While Sanskrit texts such as the Upanishads, Patanjali's Yoga Sutras, the Bhagavad Gita, *Hatha Yoga Pradipika*, and maybe the Bhagavat Purana have been largely considered as quintessential texts for yoga students, the oral traditions have by and large been ignored by multitudes of practitioners. This has amplified the elitist Brahmanical aspect of yoga, highlighting only the nivritti aspect in the ascetic-renunciate ideal or pravritti householder traditions. Both these traditions were largely patriarchal, an aspect that contemporary practitioners have not fully examined.

The spoken word was inherently disruptive of hierarchies and did not need extraneous resources for dissemination, so it existed independently outside many systems. The spoken word thrived because of practice alone due to an organic exigency generated within, rather than an imposition exerted by external systemic power. In other words, no one forced anyone to share or listen to such spontaneous utterances. Conversely, this meant that without preservation, they would be lost in the vicissitudes of time. One can surmise that while some of Mahadevi's *vachana*s or Lalla's *vakh*s are remembered and move us even today, many have been lost forever. Thus we in the modern world have to do all we can to reclaim and recenter these teachings, because they offer perspectives that are subversive, radical, and revolutionary, confronting issues of gender, conformity, religion, and caste.

If we study or consider only Sanskrit texts that are mostly from a Brahminical canon, we are missing out on an opportunity to learn from and lean into other, subaltern spiritual-philosophical perspectives and lived experiences. For any dedicated practitioner, it is prudent to listen to, learn from, or read the translations of the spoken word. Oral traditions have much to offer the world, as they are perhaps most spontaneous and hence truly personal compositions. They offer insight into the inner lives of seekers and teachers of liberation as well as the sociopolitical context of the period. This can also open doors for other inquiries into personal and cultural bias regarding the supposed superiority of the written word.

Embodiment Is Radical

Being engaged in the world as it is today, such as through social media, we are increasingly distracted and disembodied, which affects our mental, physical, and emotional health. Disembodiment, defined as "body constraints in cyberspace," is a strong predictor of "increased loneliness and depression, decreased social support, and associated with declines in psycho-social well being."[10] The antidote to disembodiment is cultivating a body-oriented, sensorial awareness of our participation, our actions, our reactions to the world around us. The embodiment practices of yoga, like asana, pranayama, mudra, and meditation, are much needed in the world today.

Bhakti poets like Akka Mahadevi worked with their whole bodies. Her nakedness was a bold statement, a fierce affirmation of her whole self—loose, unruly hair and all. It was a repudiation of any notion of shame, a revolt against what was considered respectable. It was a rejection of fear that is often associated with the physical body. She shows us that we need not cover our yearning in any way, we need not conceal our seeking for liberation. Embodiment was and is a radical idea, a rebellion against normative colonial and patriarchal constructs that thrive on compartmentalization. We are conditioned not to display our emotions, our vulnerability; we are taught that emotionality is the opposite of intellectuality, that it is weakness, that one cannot be both at the same time. Bhakti poets turned this notion on its head. Hundreds of years later, we are in a completely different world, yet we are still moved by their songs, their words, their radical unguardedness. Being in our bodies, embracing the body as it is without the need for external validation, is in itself a deeply healing and transformative practice.

Summary

Akka Mahadevi audaciously subverted patriarchal norms, asserting her rights as a seeker. She shed her clothes and her ego, and she renounced personal relationships that posed obstacles to her path of bhakti. She met many other Shiva devotees, like Basavanna and Allama Prabhu, who were also, like her, staunch critics of the caste system. Their sect, later called the Lingayats, took on many Brahmanical practices, like vegetarianism. This series of events also lends insight into the process of Sanskritization. Mahadevi's *vachana*s (spoken words) are a balm for the times we live in, filled with fire for oneness, *aikya*, and a renouncement of any form of societal stratifications.

As yoga practitioners, we aspire to cultivate insight and skill that not only tones bone, muscle, and sinew, but also hones our capacity to embody a wholeness of the human experience in all its shades and forms. Here are a few considerations for reflection:

- What are the obstacles to being embodied in our daily life? How can we shift our habits, our lifestyle, to invite more embodiment every day?

- How are these obstacles gendered or related to social hierarchies such as caste, class, race, and ability (to name a few)?

- What are the stories we tell ourselves about our bodies? What are the stories we hear about our bodies from the dominant culture?

- How can we learn from and lean into oral tradition?

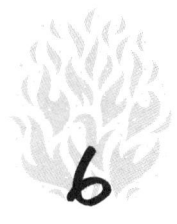

THE SONG OF PIRO

He was regal, a zoravar, *she could see that as soon as she laid eyes on him. He was a man who had power, a presence that radiated from within, anyone in his vicinity could sense that. She saw the ornate bow at his shoulder, the quiver of arrows on his back, and a sword on his hip. She recognized with a start the difference between him and his acolytes who surrounded him in the busy Lahore bazaar, fawning over every word. He was both tender and assured in his demeanor. She was not used to tenderness in men. His skin was a dusky brown; he wore an immaculately crafted turban. He was a saint, an ascetic, named Gulabdas. He beckoned her in the crowd. She, Piro, a Musalman, a Shudra, a* veshya (sex worker) *was the center of curious eyes. She stood up, diffident and yet proud. Her best friend hissed at her: Be careful, he is powerful. But she did not listen. She was overjoyed to be singled out thus. She would never forget this day, this moment. It changed her whole life.*

The memory of that day, and all that came after, came rushing in as she opened her eyes to the present. Here she was in a prison in Wazirabad, languishing so far away from her beloved guru and the dera. As she trained her eyes to the darkness around, she could see two silhouettes. Two women! Allies, she thought. Perhaps she could convince them of her innocence, perhaps they could sympathize with her sincere desire to leave worldly pleasures behind her, perhaps they would commiserate with her rejection of material attachments and understand her need to transform her wretched life. She was so steadfast in her devotion to the guru, surely they would be moved to hear about her guru, who has been a source of solace to people like her—people otherwise discarded and reviled by society. She called out to them, "O sahelis (friends), will you listen to my plea? I am sure you will agree that I have been wronged greatly, only you can save me from grave harm that will most definitely be my fate if those men return before dawn. They abducted me. You saw how they dragged me." The two women pause and listen, they were witnesses, they agreed that the men would harm her, and so they acted. They moved quickly to summon a scribe for Piro.

Piro started her letter to Gulabdas, dictating to the scribe who was hastily summoned by her new friends. She petitioned for her rescue and pleaded with the great guru for his grace, and sent the letter with a prayer. She knew in her heart that he would send help, she had complete faith in him. He had rescued her before, he would do so again. She had a dream as she lay down on the cold, hard floor: The heavy iron locks fall away, her guards are thrust aside, the doors are flung open, and she is free.

Her dream was a reality, she heard them; Gulab Singh and Chatar Singh, her guru's disciples, made such a commotion outside demanding her release. The gardener surreptitiously opened her door while the guards were thus distracted. She slipped out, and they all made haste. They rushed past the stunned guards, who followed them, shouting and cursing. The moonlit peace of the night was rudely awakened by the yelling and swearing. She ran without looking back. There were horses that awaited her! This was definitely the guru's benediction. She was astride, galloping away, hair free to the hazards of the wind and humans. She was on her way home.

The Self-Reclamation of Piro

Piro was a woman far ahead of her times, a singular woman who insisted on "agential command over her life, recording aspects of it for posterity, not to speak of the various boundaries she crossed, including the religious."[1] She was skilled in music and poetry, and her story is related in her own words in an autobiographical compilation of verses titled *Ik Sau Sath Kafian*. Through simple yet lyrical *kafis* (rhyming lines), she shares searing criticisms of the caste system and religious dogma. She sheds light on the inner workings of the Gulabdasis, an unorthodox syncretic sect, and she lets us peek into a Punjab that often was the stage for many interreligious and interdynastic conflicts. There is also an unveiling of an endearing consciousness of her gendered identity and her social status as she calls out the privilege accorded to men just on account of their gender.

Piro was born around 1832 in a Muslim Shudra family that owned land. It is believed that her arrival put an end to long years of pining, waiting, and praying. Her parents saw her as a blessed gift of the Sufi *pirs* they used to visit, and they named her Peeranditi or Peerunissa, "given by the *pirs*."[2] Piro most likely lost both her parents at an early age, and she entered a brothel around Lahore in modern Pakistan. Her verses are the most exuberant when talking about her transformative meeting with her charismatic guru, Gulabdas, and her refuge in the *dera* (a collective of people who agree upon a set of principles or doctrines). She describes the fateful meeting with Gulabdas thus:

> *Peero herself is of Khuda, filled with [divine] yearning.*
> *I saw neither Musalman nor Hindu in Him.*
> *The* pirs, *fakirs and* auliyaa*s are all entrapped,*
> *Das Gulab is beyond limits and I his* dasi.[3]

In this verse, she sees Gulabdas as the one who is beyond the limitations of religious labels, and she sees herself as one who is "of Khuda" (divine), a seeker filled with yearning for the divine. She offers herself as a *dasi*—in this context, a devoted disciple.

She was drawn to Gulabdas's radical teachings and nonconformist way of life that welcomed people from all castes, classes, genders, and religions. He was a *jnani*, who not only preached but also practiced a radical rejection of socioreligious norms. Her saga, as she recorded it, includes many dramatic events such as her abduction by her previous employer, her imprisonment, and her subsequent release, thanks to the swashbuckling soldiers/disciples sent by her guru (as narrated in my version of her story at the opening of this chapter). She also describes attempts to reconvert her to Islam by the mullahs (clergy), offers and threats that she rejected vehemently. Her *kafi*s are fueled by a bridal mysticism just like the other Bhakti poets, like Mahadevi for Shiva, except Piro's bhakti is for her guru, Gulabdas. Some scholars posit that Piro and Gulabdas were lovers,[4] a truth neither of them attempted to hide nor sought social sanction for in marriage; thus both were condemned for defying multiple norms. Piro considered him her lover as well as a divine teacher, a conduit of spiritual redemption:

> *We are neither separate, nor feel the need to merge.*
> *In an all-embracing dream we breathe,*
> *Guru-disciple fused as One.*[5]

In her *kafi*s, she often refers to herself in the first and the third person, emphasizing her sense of self, her autonomy of narrative. This emphasis is particularly poignant and powerful because women of her time and social status were not accorded agency. Patriarchy was entrenched in all the religions, classes, and castes in different ways. She was a Muslim, a Shudra, and a courtesan without any powerful patronage until she found Gulabdas. Thus, her *kafi*s are direct condemnations of men wielding enormous power in all domains, including the soteriological path that drew her into its transformative embrace. Her *kafi*s refers to all the ways in which men displayed their caste, class, and religion to assert their privilege, while women were relegated to domestic drudgery. Inspired by her guru's teachings, she rejected all outward symbols of caste and religious affiliations that keep people apart.

In one of her *kafi*s, she names all the external modes of distinction that men used from different religions, like the topknot and the thread for a Hindu, the "snipping the penis and the moustache for the Turaks" (Muslims), and the Sikh men who wear "drawers on their loins," and then she asks the bold question: What will you do with a woman, who has neither?[6] In the verses above, Piro decries these outward religious and caste distinctions that were available only to men in early nineteenth-century Punjab. While

Hindu savarna men were initiated into their jaatis with a thread (*janeu*), the women and the avarna folks were not included in these rituals of initiation. Some sects may have included women with other rituals that pointed to caste status, but by and large most women had to accept their caste standing from their association with the men in their lives. While Muslim and Sikh men also had their own specific rituals and practices that were markers of their faith, the women were on the sidelines as de facto community members. Piro's admonitions, therefore, are for men from all religious backgrounds, which informs her aspirations and motivations in joining Gulabdas, who offered succor and solace to people like her.

Piro wields a sophisticated stylistic dexterity in deploying poetic license. In her verses, she sometimes positions herself as Sita, who was captured by Ravana (her employer), and the guru who rescued her as Rama. She also displays a considerable understanding of esoteric advaita Vedantic concepts of the continuum and nonduality of consciousness and matter:

> *The body potential is sparse,*
> *the soul itself is Brahmaand/cosmos.*
> *Consider this body microcosm as the ubiquitous, all-embracing Lord.*[7]

There is also a deep yearning to belong to her new community, the Gulabdasi dera. This intrinsic need may be the reason why she not only disowns her familial Islamic roots but also calls them *mleccha*, an Indo-Vedic term that was often used in a derogatory way to refer to Muslims. It also reflects the apprehensions of a Punjab that often was the site of many power struggles between the Hindu Marathas, the Sikhs, and the Muslim Afghans and Mughal governors.

Her language in *Ik Sau Sath Kafian* is rhythmic and written in the popular Gurmukhi script. She vociferously asserts that Gulabdas is an embodiment of the divine and that the Gulabdasi dera is better than other contemporary sects. She considers herself blessed to have found refuge and solace with them, to be a part of a like-minded and like-hearted *sat-sang* (true community, or a community oriented toward the Truth). Belonging to a *sat-sang* of spiritually aligned people without hierarchical considerations was something to be grateful for, to revel in, and she did. She seems to deplore the rigidity and orthodoxy of Turak (Muslim) mullahs and the restraints of the caste system. Her whole-hearted embrace of the guru-bhakti *marga* also stemmed from egalitarian and radical aspirations, an insistence in the flattening out of differences of caste and religion. This rejection of religious affiliations is resonant with the Sikh Guru Nanak and with Kabir, the latter of whom she identified with closely because of his Muslim roots.

> *I am neither a Muslim woman, nor a Hindu,*
> *I neither accept* varnashramadharma, *nor any order's costume.*[8]

Piro never denied her courtesan life. She referred to it openly in her verses: "Keep this shelterless woman at your feet for she is a Shudra woman. . . . You who crave for love had the soiled remains." The phrase "soiled remains" is a reference to her sexual past and also displays a keen awareness of what society thought of her previous profession. She was not bound by the *pativrata* ideal of a married woman, nor did she follow the nivritti dharma as a renunciate. She was not a philosopher-*jnani*, nor was she a *tantrik* (one who practices tantra).

Piro lived in the dera for ten years and achieved the status of being regarded as "Mother," a saint of the downtrodden and the deprived.[9] Her grave was attended to with love and care. She is depicted in pictures seated on a pedestal with her guru with a follower behind them holding a *chauar* (fan), a depiction that shows respect and veneration. She was a Muslim woman, a courtesan, who lived in a dera composed predominantly of Sikh people. Piro was not from the dominant culture, class, or caste, so her very presence in the community was defiant. One can imagine the rumblings and bristlings amongst the Gulabdasis when a courtesan joined the dera. She was an outcast woman who deployed her bhakti-infused poetry with a passionate and unwavering devotion, and she came to be regarded as a "guru consort," a fierce protector of other sex workers. She transitioned from the brothel to the dera, a place of spiritual and social advancement, as a mystic.

She was an extraordinarily ordinary woman by many standards, who simply defied categorization and demanded that the world pay attention to her life and her resounding voice.

In the modern context, we may have misgivings about the intimate guru-disciple dynamic between Piro and Gulabdasi, and rightly so; there are multiple abuses of power in the religious and spiritual world (the end of the chapter explores this further). Piro, however, did not see or experience it that way. In her eyes, Gulabdas was *sat-guru*, a term that can mean someone who leads to the ultimate truth of transcendence, or someone who is a true teacher. "Piro the impure became pure on meeting the true master."[10] While there were staunch critics even then who condemned both as amoral, there were also many who witnessed and were even moved by their unconventional life and love. They were both buried in a single tomb in Chatian Wala in modern-day Pakistan.[11] Her remarkable and rebellious life and love have been kept alive through retellings of her story, like Shahryar's play *Peero Preman*, written in the Gurmukhi script, and Swarajbir's *Shairi*, dramatizations enacted both in India and Pakistan.

Piro was a woman who defied societal norms and yet yearned to belong to a community. She was sexually independent,[12] spiritually inquisitive, socially self-aware, and politically courageous. She wanted to tell her story at a time and place when, as scholar Anshu Malhotra states, "women were perhaps seen as incapable of making individual choices, and were expected to adhere to the given religious practice of their kin and community."[13] Her *kafis* reveal a depth of understanding of esoteric Upanishadic teachings of *nirguna* Brahman, while she simultaneously calls upon tales of Sita and Parvati, Puranic symbols of chaste, divine consorthood. She also remains acutely aware of her positionality and often calls herself a Shudra, a word that has multiple connotations. It points to the social status of her jaati while also alluding to the surrender of her ego in deference to her guru, a customary convention in Bhakti poetry. In doing so she aligns herself with other caste-oppressed bhakti stalwarts such as Kabir and Shabari, the tribal woman who was a devotee of Rama and who tasted fruits before offering them to him. Piro's assertion of her Shudra identity is a deft transformation of her status from that of courtesan into a devotee-consort of the guru of a dera.

The Syncretic Vision of Gulabdas

Gulabdas was a bona fide iconoclast who willfully transgressed the constructed boundaries of caste and religions, challenging many notions of societal propriety. His teachings fused tenets from multiple religions, creating his own unique blend of philosophies and practices. Born in Punjab in 1809, he most likely served as a soldier in the army. A precocious seeker, he left home at a young age and lived an itinerant life, learning from a wide array of thought traditions, from Sufi Bulleh Shah to Nath yogis to scholars of Vedanta. His thirst for truth led him to live among the naked *sadhu*s (*naga*s) and smear ash on himself. He also studied with a teacher from the Udasi tradition (a Sikh ascetic sect) before synthesizing many of these tenets and learnings to form his own Gulabdasi *sampraday* or sect within a larger tradition, a syncretic group within the Sikh community.

A fervent advocate of advaita, Gulabdas formulated a monism that included *nirguna* bhakti practiced as a reverence of the individual *jiv* (Atma) as a part of Brahman, localized within oneself. In extension of his nondualistic roots, Gulabdas identified himself as a self-realized being, Brahm, who is the divine and can lead anyone who is sincere in their spiritual aspirations. In other words, he was (and all human beings potentially were) God immanent. He espoused the path of knowledge, *jnana*, not only of philosophy but also of science (*vijnana*), and he elaborated his philosophy in his work *Gulab Chaman*. His teachings emphasized discernment (*viveka*), *birag* (*vairagya* or nonattachment), and devotion (bhakti) to the guru and the eternal truth. Using metaphorical language, he described his understanding of the interconnectedness of consciousness as God who lives within us, a truth just as real as limbs attached to a physical body:

> *Like many limbs of the body, what to speak of being close or far*
> *So god is in all, what to say of near or far.*[14]

He emphasized simplicity in both his medium of expression and his praxis. He used languages of the people—Braj, Punjabi, and Urdu—and he preached about practices like the repetition of *soham* (I am), an advaita Vedantic tenet that points to the ultimate reality of Universal Consciousness. For the Gulabdasi, *soham* was both a chant and a mantra, a practice to focus the mind as well as the vocalization of a philosophy. Just like the Sufi practice of *dhikr* (repetitive phrases of prayer) and the Sikhs' *naam simran* (remembrance of the name), *soham* was an integral aspect of the sect's praxis, a way of perpetual remembrance of the Ultimate Reality of Brahman. The aspect of nonduality also resonated with the Sufi teachings of *al-haq* (I am the Absolute Truth), which Piro elaborated in her *kafis*.

Gulabdas was not orthodox, though. He vehemently rejected the hierarchy and rigidity of varna-ashrama-dharma, and he reclaimed being an *a-jaat* (one without caste), a term sometimes used as a slur to denigrate people who either flouted casteist boundaries or were avarnas (later called Dalits). This open rebellion against the caste system was what attracted Piro and many like her. The Gulabdasi dera welcomed Muslims, Hindus, and Sikhs from all castes in all manner of appearance, with or without hair and beard (symbols of the Sikh religion).

By Gulabdas's time, Sikhism was well established in Punjab and forged its unique identity during the region's fierce struggles with the Mughal Empire. Founded by Guru Nanak in 1469 in Talwandi (in modern-day Pakistan), the religion is grounded in Guru Nanak's revelation of the infinite singular divine to be savored by everyone through their individual sensibilities.[15] The ten Sikh Gurus are an integral part of the Sikh faith, not as divine embodiments but as sacred and revered conduits. The word *Sikh* comes from the root word *shish*, meaning disciple or follower; thus, all those who followed the Guru were called Sikhs. The religion developed its own particular syntax and sacred texts, like the Sri Guru Granth Sahib, a text that contains a synthesis of the teachings of Hinduism and Islam integrated with the distinct teachings of the Gurus. Sikhs bear certain symbols of their faith, or the "five Ks" (*panj kakar* in Punjabi): uncut hair bound in a turban (*kesh*), comb (*kanga*), special undergarment (*kachaira*), iron bracelet (*kara*), and dagger (*kirpan*). Sikhism was an alternate ideological and praxis-oriented pathway for people of all caste backgrounds.

The teachings of the Gurus integrate and overlap with yoga concepts and practices, emphasizing the concepts of Oneness of Advaita Vedanta. "*Ek Onkar (AUM)*" is the first phrase in the Guru Granth Sahib. Guru Nanak emphasized the *yamas* and *niyamas* as ethical codes of behavior in the form of three precious virtues: truthfulness (*satya*), contentment (*santosha*), and surrender to divine wisdom (*ishwar-pranidhan*).[16] Bhakti and *seva* (selfless service to humanity) are inextricably linked and rooted in the notion that to serve a human is to serve the divine. There was a blending of Vedantic beliefs with Sufi vocabulary of *tauhid* (unity of being).

In addition to Sikh, Hindu, and Muslim traditions, the medieval ascetic Nath yogis (or *jogis*) also played a significant role in shaping Punjab. Founded around the eleventh century by Gorakhnath, this yogic order combined esoteric Tantra rituals with Shaivism, and they practiced hatha yoga techniques to harness physical power and spiritual prowess within and beyond the human body. While some lived on the outskirts of inhabited areas and formed monastic communities, others were more itinerant, traveling great distances, while still others were "warrior ascetics," an umbrella term for armed ascetics or *sanyasis* (an earlier name was the *naga*, from the Sanskrit word *nanga*, meaning naked). The *sanyasis* or *jogis* came from different Bhakti sects—the Shaiva and Vaishnava—and gained prominence in the 1500s. Warrior asceticism was not confined to "Hindu" traditions; the Sufi fakirs also banded together with "state of the art weaponry, [and] knew how to use it; they were unruly, hardy ascetics with little regard for state authority."[17] Gulabdas lived among the heterodox and radical Nath yogis for a while and was influenced by their teachings.

Sikhism attracted a large following in Punjab with its monotheistic, egalitarian, and secular teachings, much to the consternation of Aurangzeb, the Mughal king (1658–1707). Aurangzeb was unlike his predecessor, the liberal-minded Akbar, who had abolished the *jaziya* (a military tax for non-Muslims) and founded an interreligious Din-Ilahi (Divine Faith) integrating tenets from Islam and Vedanta. Aurangzeb was driven by Islamic orthodoxy and clashed often with his brother Dara Shikoh (whom Aurangzeb eventually had killed), who sponsored the translations of the Upanishads. He also ordered the beheading of the ninth Sikh guru, Guru Tegh Bahadur. Thus, under the stewardship of Guru Gobind Singh, Sikhism also integrated a robust militaristic stream, the Khalsa, generated as a response to the Islamic orthodox oppression of Aurangzeb. The Khalsa were a disciplined body of saints and soldiers, men and women of courage who adhered to the strictest codes of conduct and the highest morality.[18]

Gulabdas's Punjab was one of the epicenters of many religious and political cross-currents. Gulabdasis were inheritors of shared religious traditions, religiosities expressed in idioms that were specific to their own theological orientation.[19] Thus, the Gulabdasi dera blossomed at a time when syncretism and heterodoxy was on the rise in Punjab. In addition to rejecting religious boundaries, Gulabdas accepted somewhat hedonistic (for his times) practices, like mixing genders in the dera and openly being seen in the company of sex workers. He also had intimate relationships with a few other women, including Piro, without marriage.[20]

While Sikhism subscribed to the path of the "ascetic householder" and had celibate as well as householder followers, Gulabdas repudiated the necessity of celibacy and marriage as well as the garb of the typical ascetic. Instead he practiced and preached "*jog* and *bhog*," i.e., yoga (nonattachment) and enjoyment or pleasure, much to the criticism and dismay of more orthodox Hindu, Muslim, and Sikh teachers. Many of his followers were young, influential, and wealthy. He was a teacher of the soldiers of King Ranjit Singh's army, which may be one of the reasons why his Gulabdasi dera could live without much censorship in the Punjab of the mid-1800s.

Gulabdas was considered a *sant*, a word that is sometimes wrongly translated as "saint." *Sant* comes from the Sanskrit root word *san*, meaning truth or essence. A *sant* is regarded as a being who has attained moksha or spiritual enlightenment, who can guide the seeker in their quest for the ultimate truth of the Self. Inspired and informed by Sikh *sant*-guru traditions and his own explorations of Vedanta, Sufi, and Nath yogi teachings, Gulabdas charted his own spiritual path, welcoming people from all caste and religious backgrounds. Even in his last moments, Gulabdas resisted convention in a telling move that proclaimed his love for and intimacy with Piro: He defied the traditions of cremation and left instructions that he was to be buried together with her in the same tomb.

Key Takeaways

The Complexity of Syncretism and Hybridization

Syncretism is the negotiation and interaction of elements that stem from essentially different groups or domains into one particular group or domain; it signifies the heterogeneity of historical processes as opposed to an idealized homogeneity.[21] Religious syncretism occurs when there are interactions between different belief systems that lead to the synthesis of a new one. Few religions are completely untouched by elements of other religions; most have layers and strands from other religions.

There are many dimensions and aspects of syncretism, especially in terms of power, dominance, and control. Religion was one of the main tools to assert authority, and colonizers weaponized it. Syncretism could also aid expansion, such as the Buddhist integration of regional customs when spreading through Asia; or it could be a creative response to the colonizing culture imposing values, belief systems, habits, and customs upon the colonized. Thus, syncretism could also counter the homogenizing tendencies of imperialism. For instance, Gulabdas founded his dera upon an integration of elements of all three major religious traditions of Punjab—Hinduism, Sikhism, and Sufism—and a rejection of the essentialism and authority of any one religion. He carved out a spacious container to hold only what nourished and supported all participants while pushing at the seams of oppositional and rigid religious boundaries.

Syncretism is not free from criticism. Human beings have an intrinsic need to belong to something definite or "pure," whether a culture, a religion, or a tradition; we tend to be apprehensive of ambiguity. However, all religions have evolved and changed and are dynamic processes rather than static products. In addition, there is also a concern about the locus of power, i.e., the dominant culture gets to fuse elements from different traditions and determine what is chosen in the processes of syncretism. At a time when we are chastened by impositions of various compartmentalizations, the fluidity between religions and the merging of varied belief systems are important reminders for contemporary times.

Syncretism and hybridization are not new to yoga. Yoga is accretive, with layers and iterations further developing a particular idea or critiquing some aspect. The Upanishads were iterations of the Vedas; the bhakti and Tantra traditions emerged as a challenge to Brahmanical orthodoxy. Hatha yoga practices were enriched by a Tantric understanding of the gross and subtle bodies. There was a dynamic discarding or integration of elements of belief systems and practices. Yoga has been shaped by religious, sociopolitical, and economic factors. Caste and gender, and later colonialism and capitalism, were also important factors in the development of modern yoga. Thus, the questions we should consider when discussing cultural appropriation need to expand to regard historical and current loci of power and influence in yoga—dominant caste, class, race, and gender.

The Contested Place of the Guru in Yoga

The guru has had an exalted space in almost all yoga and other ancient South Asian traditions. More than a teacher or an instructor, a guru has experiential wisdom and has been revered as a person who leads one to the light within. The guru-disciple relationship has a long history, especially because the teachings were originally oral transmissions; thus, narrations and instructions needed to be preserved intact. During ancient times, a guru (maybe a householder, an ascetic, or both) accepted disciples (*shishya*) into the *gurukul* (residence schools), often on the outskirts of towns, where they lived together in a somewhat reciprocal relationship.

A guru would share the wisdom and knowledge of various texts and/ or guide the *shishya* in learning rituals and skills that were deemed important according to their varna. The student had to help out with running the *gurukul* and serve the teacher and his family. The gurus were mostly men during the Vedic period and the heyday of the Tantra traditions (see chapter 3). The Vedas and the Upanishads contain exaltations and idealizations of the guru as the dispeller of darkness:

> *The syllable* gu *means darkness, the syllable* ru, *he who dispels it*
> *Because of the power to dispel darkness, the guru is thus named.*
>
> —*Advayataraka Upanishad, verse 16*[22]

The Buddhist and Jain traditions regard the role of the guru as paramount to one's spiritual journey. Many Tantra lineages (*sampradays*) center the role of the guru as a pivotal figure, one who initiates the *sadhaka* or *sadhaki* into the path, a most important primary step before the commencement of any of the other rituals and practices. Sikh gurus are revered as primary conduits of spiritual wisdom. Each guru is considered as a manifestation of Guru Nanak, the vessel (*mahal*) of the same consciousness.

The place of the guru is also fraught with embedded inequalities and imbalances of power from the perspectives of both caste and gender. This dynamic is mentioned in epics like the Mahabharata (see chapter 3). In a more modern context, most of the influential gurus of yoga traditions have been savarna men. Many of them have grossly misused and abused power in overt, covert, and violent ways. I name only a few to highlight the degree and prevalence of gross violation in yoga spaces—places and practices that are considered to be healing and liberatory. This list is by no means exhaustive. Pattabhi Jois, the influential teacher of the Ashtanga school of yoga; Bikram Chowdhury, the millionaire yoga entrepreneur who popularized "hot yoga"; Satchidananda, founder of Integral Yoga; Yogi Bhajan (also known as Harbhajan Singh Khalsa), the founder of Kundalini Yoga; and so many others have been accused of sexual misconduct by hundreds of women.[23] While each of the women have their distinct experiences of abuse or assault, an overarching thread runs through their stories. There is an embedded power difference in the relationship between the guru and the disciple-student. In addition, institutional hierarchy enacted by people close to the guru ensures silence when women speak up about abuse.

The guru's place in the spiritual journey is a sacred one, and if we are very fortunate, we may come across someone who sees our light. As yoga practitioners in today's world, we also need to be cognizant of structural power in a yoga space, and we must be discerning about who we learn from. Perhaps we need to begin noticing who we quote on a regular basis and who we are drawn to, and ensure we learn from a wide array of teachers and philosophies.

The contributions of women and gender-expansive folks, avarna traditions, and heterodox streams are not as well-known or are sometimes completely disregarded in yogic studies and praxis. Even today, most people still center and quote primarily Brahmin men. Perhaps we can hold on to the *guru tattva*, the essence of the teacher, the lineage, and the teachings,[24] and ensure that deification of the teacher doesn't overcome critical thinking. This may be a challenging thing to do, especially since the guru holds a revered position in many yoga traditions; yet it can also be a liberatory practice. By tugging at a thread of power in yoga, there is an intentional unraveling of the convoluted and unnamed hierarchies of caste, gender, race, abilities, and class that also operate in other dimensions. Thus, cultivating discernment about yoga teachers and gurus can be an integral step in dismantling structural oppression.

Here are some questions for reflection:

- How can you deploy radical imagination as a subversion of hegemony?

- A *sat-sang*, like Piro's dera, can be a space for radical imagination. How can you cocreate a loving, inclusive, and disruptive *sat-sang*?

- What are the qualities you look for in your teacher-guru? Have they shifted in any way?

Summary

Piro's life is a rich study in contradictions and complexities. She is an avid devotee as well as a rebellious dissenter. As a renegade Shudra Muslim courtesan who escapes her captors, she then chooses to be a part of a somewhat cloistered Sikh-Hindu monastic dera. Her deployment of bhakti and alignment with Kabir and Shabari is an expression of her intuitive and strategic self-identification as a rebel who is also a devoted spiritual aspirant. Her *kafis* seamlessly integrate elements of advaita monism with Sikh and Sufi traditions as she skillfully uses dramatic and metaphorical language to compare herself to Sita abducted by Ravana, waiting to be rescued by her Rama (Gulabdas). Her fiercely independent voice is a ferocious critic of religious dogma, and at the same time, she is a *dasi* (devotee-student) to her charismatic and influential *zoravar*. Gulabdas's syncretic dera, which rejected the constraints of varna-ashrama-dharma, made it possible for Piro and others like her to locate both a refuge and a container in which creative resistance could find a loving place.

Conclusion
Embodied Resistance

A few wild ideas animate this book. Although there may be differences within the vast and complex yoga tapestry, these musings are a crystallization of some of the core teachings of yoga: that we are not separate from each other, that each one of us is an embodiment of consciousness, and that we are a vital part of all of creation. Yoga unveils this *prajna*, the realization that the Self is beyond the limitations of mind-body conditioning. A corollary to this teaching is *avidya* (ignorance of inherent interconnectedness), which builds systems and institutions that keep us in perennial hierarchies. Caste, race, gender, and class are human creations, not divine ordinations. Liberation is the dismantling and dissolution of constructs that ossify all of us into narrow understandings of the expanse of human potential.

The second idea is that of interdependence among all of creation. There is an overarching emphasis on reciprocity in yoga: Every act, every thought, every action has consequences and leaves an imprint, not only on our own individual psyches, generating *samskara*s, but also on the interweaving threads that connect us to each other. Interconnectedness also means there is an interdependence so that when someone is hurt, needs support or rest, the other picks up the load one way or the other. The sramanas who renounced all attachment to the material world were also in connection with the community. The Buddhist *bhikku*s or monks went from home to home, accepting offerings of food from people from all caste and class backgrounds. In exchange, they taught and shared the teachings of Buddha and the *dhamma*, the moral and spiritual path to enlightenment. The teachings for householder-practitioners were rooted in notions of mutual dependence, that one cannot turn away from responsibilities to the other.

The last and perhaps most integral idea is that we do not perfect transformation; we practice transformation. *Abhyasa* (practice) is the unit of change, both on and off the mat. Thus, if we aim to cocreate a just and loving world, we have to practice our orientations toward justice and liberation; we have to "do" the loving as courageous disruption of the oppressions of the status quo.

The planet is in peril. Ecological disasters, genocides, and wars abound. There is not only a rise in authoritarian regimes around the world, but also an active support of authoritarian governments and figures. A recent study found that among the populations of twenty-four nations, more than 31 percent of the people overall supported some form of authoritarian government.[1] The world we know and live in is ablaze with nationalisms, racism, casteism, religious fundamentalism, homophobia, transphobia, and misogyny. The far right in India and the far right in the United States are colluding in dangerous ways. In an October 2020 survey, most Indians located in India who supported the Hindu nationalist political party Bharatiya Janata Party also professed support for Donald Trump's blatant white supremacism.[2] In diasporic locations like the United States, Hindutva organizations—despite representing minority communities—"work in concert with other far-right actors to advance an anti-democratic politics where the civil rights and religious freedoms of Hindus are framed in opposition to, and at the expense of, those of other communities."[3] Caste continues to be present in the diaspora. Per a 2016 report from Equality Labs, 67 percent of Dalits surveyed in the diaspora reported being treated unfairly at their workplace because of their caste; 12 percent of Shudras report the same. Approximately 40 percent of Dalit respondents and 14 percent of Shudra respondents reported that they were made to feel unwelcome at their place of worship because of their caste.[4] This data extended over a spectrum of religions, including Hindu temples, Sikh gurudwaras, churches, and mosques.

Yoga spaces are a microcosm of larger social, political, and economic systems and institutions. Yoga has been and is weaponized in nationalist movements and ideologies. The previous chapters shared glimpses into the interweaving threads of Brahmanism, hegemony, and patriarchy in the tapestry of yoga. The need of the times is not only to unravel these interwoven strands and understand the sociohistorical context of the teachings but also to investigate how the teachings have been institutionalized and internalized as core values and absolute truths. From dharma to karma, from the demonization of the "other" in epics to the notion that Sanskrit is the root language of yoga, from the historical appropriation of regional and village deities to the assertions of pristineness of the past, yoga practitioners need to examine the corpus of yoga relative to our specific and unique positionalities. As a savarna, this excavation is an ongoing inquiry.

Yoga is not apolitical. It never has been. The myriad roots of yoga also lie in a radical rejection of ritualism and Brahmanical hegemony. The tension between heterodoxy and orthodoxy is a vital part of yoga history. History teaches us that resistance comes in many shapes, textures, and forms. There were those who discarded all religious dogma, like Kabir, and those who syncretized different elements of religions, like Gulabdas. There were those who broke through the boundaries of caste and gender, like Janabai and Kanaka, and those who picked up swords and fought rival factions of warrior-yogis.

In each of the stories—from Sulabha, who questioned the spiritual and intellectual prowess of a powerful king, to Radha with her full-bodied, wholehearted searing love, to Piro, who unabashedly insisted that her story had value and relevance, to Akka Mahadevi, who shed her clothes and all other patriarchal notions of propriety—there have been rebellious voices that have vociferously claimed their place in the constellation of changemakers. Their voices can light up our own paths to healing and transformation, at the individual and systemic levels. To continue your explorations of the core concepts of this book, next I offer some recommendations for how to RISE—Root, Integrate, Study, and take Embodied Action—in the hope that this sparks your own critical inquiries as yoga practitioners.

Root: Just as the vitality of a tree lies in the robustness of the roots, each one of us, as yoga practitioners, can know and understand our own roots, the many truths of our ancestors. Being rooted, grounded in self-knowledge and self awareness, is key to discerning how we can act with integrity. The unearthing of complex histories is a necessary, ongoing excavation of multiple truths. In the specific context of modern yoga, white supremacy is manifested in multiple ways, from xenophobia to the erasure of Black, South Asian, and other marginalized communities. Reductiveness of the practice is a function of white supremacy and neoliberal spiritual capitalism. While this needs to be challenged, there is also a need to challenge historical appropriation from Indigenous and tribal traditions and to acknowledge the Brahmanization in yoga that happened over centuries.

Appreciation and appropriation are not binaries; they exist in context of caste, class, race, and gender. The emphasis on Sanskrit as the original language of yoga is simplistic. Sanskrit is an ancestral language for many South Asians, along with other ancient languages like Pali and Prakrit. Sanskrit has never been accessible to caste-oppressed communities, so including texts and books from regional languages can broaden and deepen study and perspective.

In order to cocreate welcoming yoga spaces that can nourish people from all lived experiences, each of us has a role to play according to our own lived experience and positionality of caste, class, race, ability, and gender. As savarna yoga practitioners and teachers, cocreation of spaces that hold complexities is an important step in the acknowledgement of the history of caste oppression, especially centering the lived experiences and expertise of caste-oppressed folks. As a cis savarna woman who shares the teachings of yoga, I acknowledge my own privilege, and I collaborate with teachers from other lived experiences and expertise. As a brown woman in a white (yoga) world, I also have experienced erasure and racism. This is an invitation for white yoga practitioners to unravel their ancestry and the ways in which solidarity with folks from marginalized communities can be an ongoing practice.

Integrate: Taking time to integrate and synthesize new learnings is a vital and often underemphasized aspect of transformation. We live in a world that needs quick fixes and rapid closure, demanding our attention on multiple things simultaneously. Unraveling deeply rooted intergenerational biases and trauma is a lifelong process. Spiritual consumerism plays an integral role in neoliberal capitalism. There is an overselling of everything from yoga apparel to workshops to retreats as Band-Aids for healing deeper wounds inflicted by multiple structural oppressions. Internalizing new learnings—and, perhaps more importantly, unlearning the old ones—entails slowing down and introspection.

Study: Study history from multiple sources and from diverse lived experiences. Who are the authors and teachers you often quote? Are they from a particular caste, race, class, and/or gender? We often gravitate toward worldviews that confirm our own. It is challenging to listen to, read, or study folks who have diametrically different perspectives or who confront our own notion of an unsullied and pristine ancestry. And yet, this is vital in the path toward fostering a practice of radical disruption.

It will take a lifetime of dedicated study (and then some) to gain a deep understanding of yoga. To return to the metaphor of the tree, study is equivalent to nourishment, so you need a variety of sources to ensure the tree's optimal health, resilience, and longevity. Ensuring that sources of study come from varied frames of reference and backgrounds is important to prevent insularity of community and thought.

Embodied action: Most importantly, yoga is about practice. As Dr. Angela Davis said in a panel discussion about the nature and role of practice, "Our practices on the mat, on the cushion are rehearsals for living, for revolution, for abolition. We explore aspects and dimensions of freedoms that we did not know ever existed."[5]

While it is imperative to study and integrate, it is also important for us to act with our whole selves, with self-awareness, intention, care, and skill. Most people are either burned out, in denial, or overwhelmed at the state of the world. Yet act we must, in big ways and small. Yoga offers us many pathways into embodiment, from asana to pranayama to sangha. As yoga practitioners we practice being with discomfort, and we learn our ways into ease and rest.

Embodied action is unique and specific, and is shaped by one's skill and lived experience. It can involve connecting people and resources, sharing and donating to mutual aid efforts, or leveraging privilege in a yoga group to include and center marginalized voices. It can consist of frontline organizing in communities of influence or participating in education and campaign efforts organized by antioppression groups. What if we reimagine our yoga community as mindful agents of social change and practice yoga as active, embodied resistance to systems of oppression?

The breath of history lives on in us, in our cultural memories. The stories in this book are a hopeful ode to resistance and emancipation of all, in yoga spaces and beyond, shedding light on the paths chosen by our ancestors: debate, dissent, spoken word, radical love, and a rebellious discarding of the shackles of patriarchal norms. What would these paths of resistance look like in today's world? How can we unravel the threads of dominance and hegemony that run through the tapestry of yoga? How can we cocreate communities that can hold multiplicities, dissent, and conflict? These are the questions we need to ponder and then act upon with dedication and radical love. I hope this work inspires you to ask brave questions, to hold space for complexity and multiple truths, to seek the story of a story and the many truths of a word. I hope these stories of extraordinary and ordinary folks light up your path toward a reclamation of yoga as embodied resistance—as an ongoing practice of collective care and liberation. Resistance is a rejection of normalization of oppression. Resistance is a vociferous proclamation of the agency and sovereignty of all human beings, not just some. Resistance is a practice rooted in reenvisioning traditions and paradigms that entrench historical and contemporary hierarchies. As Thenmozhi articulates in the foreword, integrative practice is our birthright. It is time to remember and then act.

The time is now.

Glossary

Adivasi: Collective term for the Indigenous peoples of South Asia; *adi*: from the beginning; *vasi*: inhabitants.

advaita: Nondualism or nonsecondness; the individual principle (Atma) is identical with infinite being (Brahman).

Atma: The individual principle, or Self; Hindu and Jain conceptualization.

avarnas: Heterogeneous groups of people who are not a part of the four varnas (i.e., Dalits and Adivasis).

Brahman: Eternal consciousness or infinite being (from the Upanishads, in the Vedas).

Brahmana: Texts on Vedic rituals.

Brahmin: Scholar or priest.

Dalit: Marathi word for "scattered, broken." In the 1880s activist and social reformer Jyotirao Phule used this term to refer to people outside the varna system who were until then referred to as "untouchables" by people within the varna system.

***darshana*:** From *drs-*, to see. It can mean the auspicious viewing of a deity or a perspective/philosophical viewpoint.

Dasa: Slave or servant; outsider or non-Vedic people; also has been used to refer to *bhakta*: servant of a deity.

dera: Domicile of doctrinally like-minded people. More popularly referred to as a sect.

dvaita: From *dvi-*, two; the theological premise that two principles or realities can exist simultaneously; Self and Brahman are distinct.

fakir: Mendicant or renunciate, usually referring to a Sufi ascetic.

godhadi: Quilt or tapestry.

guna: Attribute, quality, or characteristic. There are three *guna*s in the Samkhya system: *sattva*, *rajas*, and *tamas*.

jaati: Endogamous groups; colloquially called a caste.

jnana: Knowledge or gnosis.

karma: Action; from a Vedic perspective, it means ritual action. The karma yoga of the Gita refers to yoga of action, which means doing one's duties per one's varna, without attachment to the outcome.

kathaka: Storyteller.

Kshatriya: Ruler or warrior class of the varna system.

mleccha: From Vedic Sanskrit referring to the non-Aryan people; also refers to "foreigners" like the Huns, Mongols, Turks, Kushans, and many others.

prakriti: Nature; creative force; active element of the universe.

pooja: Ceremonial worship; offerings of flowers or fruits.

punya: Virtue or merit. In Hinduism, performing virtuous actions determined by one's varna in this birth is considered to benefit the next. The Buddhist understanding of *punya* is that which confers happiness.

Puranas: Meaning old or ancient; texts of myths, legends, and lore covering a range of topics, including the nature of the universe, genealogies of gods and goddesses, love stories, hagiographies of sages, astronomy, and so on. The Puranas are from Jain and Hindu traditions and are named after the major deities of the pantheon, like Vishnu, Shiva, and Mahadevi. Puranas synthesize Vedic thought as well as the later bhakti streams.

purusa: Undifferentiated consciousness of the Samkhya philosophy; an entity corresponding to the concept of Brahman of Upanishadic literature.

*rajas***:** *Guna* or attribute of dynamism or action.

*sadhana***:** Discipline or practice for the attainment of goals, either salvation or *siddhi*s. Tantric *sadhana* requires initiation and guidance from a guru.

Samkhya: Literally meaning "enumeration"; the philosophical system that undergirds many of the yoga texts, like the Yoga Sutras of Patanjali. It posits a multiplicity of entities: purusa (undifferentiated consciousness) and prakriti (the material-phenomenal aspect of reality).

samsara: The phenomenal or material world; also refers to the endless cycles of birth and death.

*samskara***:** Deeply embedded or inherited psychological-physical patterns or imprints.

savarnas: Members of the four varnas.

*shishya***:** Disciple.

Shudra: The fourth (and oppressed) category of the varnas; laborers and artisans of the later Vedic period.

*siddhi***:** Knowledge or accomplishment; also refers to miraculous powers or paranormal capabilities gained by Tantric or yogic *sadhana*s.

Upanishads: Texts that distilled Vedic rituals, elaborating key philosophical and ontological tenets of the Vedas.

Vaishya: Varna of agriculturists, moneylenders, and traders.

varna: Meaning ranges across color, order, and class. Social stratification system with four hierarchically ranked classes: Brahmins, Kshatriyas, Vaishyas, and Shudras. Adivasis and Dalits are avarna.

Vedanta: Literal meaning: end of the Vedas or the culmination of Vedic knowledge. The Upanishads and the Gita are referred to as Vedanta.

Vedas: From *vid*, to know or comprehend. Repositories of knowledge composed in Vedic Sanskrit. There are four Vedas: Rig, Sama, Yajur, and Atharva. Each Veda has four components or layers: Brahmana (commentaries on rituals and sacrifices or the *yajnas*), Samhita (benedictions and mantras), Aranyaka (meanings of rituals), and Upanishad (philosophies and rituals). Also elaborates on the *chaturvarna* (four varnas).

yuga: Period or unit of time. Each *yuga* is progressively shorter than the previous one. Four such *yuga*s (called Krita, Treta, Dvapara, and the present Kali) make up the *mahayuga* ("great *yuga*").

Notes

Introduction

1 Romila Thapar, *The Future in the Past: Essays and Reflections* (Aleph Book Company, 2023).

2 Soutik Biswas, "Oppenheimer: How He Was Influenced by the Bhagavad Gita," *BBC*, July 24, 2023, https://www.bbc.com/news/world-asia-india-66288900.

3 Gerda Lerner, *Living with History/Making Social Change* (University of North Carolina Press, 2009), 164.

4 Andrea R. Jain, *Peace Love Yoga: The Politics of Global Spirituality* (Oxford Academic, 2020), 43.

5 Jain, *Peace Love Yoga*, 43.

6 Jain, *Peace Love Yoga*, 77.

7 Jain, *Peace Love Yoga*.

8 Patanjali Group, accessed February 28, 2025, https://patanjali.group/.

9 HT Correspondent, "Ramdev Offers to 'Cure Homosexuals' at His Haridwar Ashram," *Hindustan Times*, December 11, 2013, https://www.hindustantimes.com/india/ramdev-offers-to-cure-homosexuals-at-his-haridwar-ashram/story-UtnktIHM8qAdT5NKbG7QsO.html.

10 Prashant Waikar, "Reading Islamophobia in Hindutva: An Analysis of Narendra Modi's Political Discourse," *Islamophobia Studies Journal* 4, no. 2 (2018): 161–80, https://doi.org/10.13169/islastudj.4.2.0161.

11 "Vision and Mission," Rashtriya Swayamsevak Sangh, March 13, 2015, https://www.rss.org//Encyc/2015/3/13/Vision-and-Mission.html.

12 Mrinal Pande, "Gendered Analysis of Hindutva Imaginaries: Manipulation of Symbols for Ethnonationalist Projects," *Journal of Modern European History* 20, no. 3 (2022): 4, https://doi.org/10.1177/16118944221110725.

13 Narendra Modi, "Statement by H. E. Narendra Modi, Prime Minister of India," General Debate of the 69th Session of the United Nations General Assembly, New

York, September 27, 2014, https://www.un.org/en/ga/69/meetings/gadebate/pdf/IN_en.pdf.

14 "International Day of Yoga 21 June," United Nations, accessed February 26, 2025, https://www.un.org/en/observances/yoga-day.

15 Rhea Mogul, "Modi's Muslim Remarks Spark 'Hate Speech' Accusations as India's Mammoth Election Deepens Divides," *CNN*, April 22, 2024, https://www.cnn.com/2024/04/22/asia/india-modi-muslim-hate-speech-allegations-intl-hnk/index.html.

16 Ian Vásquez et al. *The Human Freedom Index 2023: A Global Measurement of Personal, Civic, and Economic Freedom* (Cato Institute and Fraser Institute, 2023), https://www.cato.org/human-freedom-index/2023.

17 "Human Freedom Index," Cato Institute, 2024, https://www.cato.org/human-freedom-index/2024.

18 Amnesty International, "India: Authorities Must End Repression of Dissent in Jammu and Kashmir," Amnesty International, September 18, 2024, https://www.amnesty.org/en/latest/news/2024/09/india-authorities-must-end-repression-of-dissent-in-jammu-and-kashmir/.

19 Sheena Sood, "Om-Washing: Why Modi's Yoga Day Pose Is Deceptive," *Al Jazeera*, June 22, 2023, https://www.aljazeera.com/opinions/2023/6/22/om-washing-modis-yoga-day-pose-of-deception.

20 Deeksha Udupa and Raqib Hameed Naik, "The Hindu Nationalist Campaign to Promote Yoga," *The Nation*, April 6, 2023, https://www.thenation.com/article/culture/yogathon-hindu-nationalism/.

21 "The Hindu Roots of Yoga," Hindu American Foundation, accessed March 4, 2025, https://www.hinduamerican.org/projects/hindu-roots-of-yoga.

22 Krishnadev Calamur, "Calif. Judge Rules Yoga in Public Schools Not Religious," *NPR*, July 1, 2013, https://www.npr.org/sections/thetwo-way/2013/07/01/197712791/calif-judge-rules-yoga-in-public-schools-not-religious.

23 Amartya Sen, *The Argumentative Indian* (Picador, 2006).

24 Thapar, *Essays and Reflections*.

25 Tracy Pintchman, *The Rise of the Goddess in the Hindu Tradition* (SUNY Press, 1994), 2.

26 Arti Dhand, *Woman as Fire, Woman as Sage: Sexual Ideology in the Mahābhārata* (SUNY Press, 2009), 17.

27 Tristan Katz (@tristankatzcreative), "Additionally, I wonder if folks consider non-binary and genderfluid individuals when using womxn and women+," Instagram, November 18, 2024, https://www.instagram.com/p/DChRIUevVly/?img_index=6&igsh=MzRlODBiNWFlZA==.

28 A. K. Ramanujan, *The Collected Essays of A. K. Ramanujan* (Oxford University Press, 1999).

29 Alf Hiltebeitel, *The Cult of Draupadi: Mythologies From Gingee to Kurukshetra*, vol. 1 (University of Chicago Press, 1991).

30 Rita D. Sherma, introduction to *Hermeneutics and Hindu Thought: Toward a Fusion of Horizons*, ed. Rita D. Sherma and Arvind Sharma (Springer, 2008), 3.

Chapter 1: Origins of Yoga and Hinduism

1 Nistula Hebbar, "Rig Veda Golden Age for Women's Rights: Sangh History Body," *The Hindu*, September 20, 2015, https://www.thehindu.com/news/national/rig-veda-golden-age-for-womens-rights-sangh-history-body/article7669178.ece.

2 Tony Joseph, *Early Indians: The Story of Our Ancestors and Where We Came From* (Juggernaut, 2018).

3 Joseph, *Early Indians*.

4 Wendy Doniger, *The Hindus: An Alternative History* (Penguin Classics, 2009), 67.

5 Abraham Eraly, *Gem in the Lotus: The Seeding of Indian Civilisation* (Penguin Books India, 2000), 35.

6 Franklin Southworth and David McAlpin, "30 South Asia: Dravidian Linguistic History," *The Encyclopedia of Global Human Migration*, February 4, 2013, https://doi.org/10.1002/9781444351071.wbeghm830.

7 Doniger, *The Hindus*.

8 Doniger, *The Hindus*.

9 David Kinsley, *Hindu Goddesses: Visions of the Divine Feminine in the Hindu Religious Traditions* (University of California Press, 1988).

10 D. N. Jha, *The Myth of the Holy Cow* (Verso, 2002), 30.

11 Jha, *The Myth of the Holy Cow*, 20.

12 "Violent Cow Protection in India," Human Rights Watch, February 18, 2019, https://www.hrw.org/report/2019/02/19/violent-cow-protection-india/vigilante-groups-attack-minorities.

13 Romila Thapar, *A History of India: Volume 1* (Penguin Books, 1990), 39–40.

14 Doniger, *The Hindus*.

15 Thapar, *A History of India*.

16 Gail Omvedt, *Understanding Caste: From Buddha to Ambedkar and Beyond* (Orient Black Swan, 2012).

17 Thapar, *A History of India*, 62.

18 Arti Dhand, *Woman as Fire, Woman as Sage: Sexual Ideology in the Mahābhārata* (SUNY Press, 2009).

19 Doniger, *The Hindus*, 103.

20 Thapar, *A History of India*, 46.

21 Tracy Pintchman, *The Rise of the Goddess in the Hindu Tradition* (SUNY Press, 1994).

22 Uma Chakravarti, *Gendering Caste: Through a Feminist Lens* (Sage Publications, 2018), 11.

23 Bhimrao Ambedkar, *Annihilation of Caste: The Annotated Critical Edition* (Verso, 2016), 233.

24 Thenmozhi Soundararajan, *The Trauma of Caste: A Dalit Feminist Meditation on Survivorship, Healing, and Abolition* (North Atlantic Books, 2022), 45.

25 Thapar, *A History of India*, 51.

26 Thapar, *A History of India*.

27 Omvedt, *Understanding Caste*, 12.

28 Omvedt, *Understanding Caste*, 12.

29 Pupul Jayakar, *The Earthen Drum* (National Museum of Delhi, 1980), 6.

30 Pintchman, *The Rise of the Goddess*.

31 Pintchman, *The Rise of the Goddess*, 12.

32 Pintchman, *The Rise of the Goddess*, 11.

33 Doniger, *The Hindus*.

34 Bibek Debroy, *Valmiki Ramayana* (India Penguin Classics, 2017), xi.

Chapter 2: Is Yoga Hindu?

1 Rakhi Sharma (@_spiritual_therapy), "Hindu push-ups For Beginners," Instagram, June 28, 2024, https://www.instagram.com/reel/C8wryNOPnlN/?igsh =NTc4MTIwNjQ2YQ==.

2 Wendy Doniger and B. K. Smith, trans., *The Laws of Manu* (Penguin Classics, 1991), 19.

3 Bhimrao Ambedkar, *Annihilation of Caste: The Annotated Critical Edition* (Verso, 2016), 241–42.

4 Sunanda K. Datta Ray, "Secularism Is the Core Safeguard India Needs," *Deccan Chronicle*, December 31, 2018, https://www.deccanchronicle.com/opinion /columnists/010119/secularism-is-the-core-safeguard-india-needs.html.

5 Gurcharan Das, *The Difficulty of Being Good: On the Subtle Art of Dharma* (Oxford University Press, 2010), 306.

6 Das, *The Difficulty of Being Good*.

7 Das, *The Difficulty of Being Good*.

8 R. Mahalaksmi, "Sanatana Dharma's Historical Roots Reveal a Complex Journey," *Frontline*, October 5, 2023, https://frontline.thehindu.com/the-nation/essay
-r-mahalakshmi-on-sanatana-dharma-historical-interpretations-contemporary
-concerns-roots-reveal-a-complex-journey/article67326266.ece.

9 Mahalaksmi, "Sanatana Dharma's Historical Roots."

10 Mahalaksmi, "Sanatana Dharma's Historical Roots."

11 Ambedkar, quoted in Ankur Barua and Vishal Vasanthakumar, "Renaming Caste,
Retaining Privilege," *The India Forum*, June 15, 2024, https://www.theindiaforum
.in/caste/renaming-caste-retaining-privilege.

12 David Lorenzen, "Who Invented Hinduism?," *Comparative Studies in Society and
History* 41, no. 4 (1999): 630–59, https://doi.org/10.1017/S0010417599003084.

13 Lorenzen, "Who Invented Hinduism?," 646.

14 Lorenzen, "Who Invented Hinduism?," 651.

15 Tanvir Anjum, "The Emergence of Muslim Rule in India: Some Historical Disconnects and Missing Links," *Islamic Studies* 46, no. 2 (2007): 217, https://www
.jstor.org/stable/20839068.

16 Manu Pillai, "A Mosque Celebrating a Hindu King," *Manu S. Pillai* (blog),
November 14, 2019, https://manuspillai.com/2019/11/14/a-mosque-celebrating
-a-hindu-king-16-november-2019/.

17 Audrey Truschke, *Culture of Encounters: Sanskrit at the Mughal Court* (Penguin
Random House India, 2017), 13.

18 Azeez Tharuvana, *Living Ramayanas: Exploring the Plurality of the Epic in
Wayanad and the World* (Eka, 2021).

19 Carl Ernst, *Refractions of Islam in India: Situating Sufism and Yoga* (Sage Publications, 2016).

20 Veronique Bouillier, "Aurangzeb and the Nāth Yogīs," *Journal of the Royal Asiatic
Society* 28, no. 3 (2018): 525–35, https://doi.org/10.1017/S1356186318000081.

21 Sharada Sugirtharajah, "Max Mueller and Textual Management: A Postcolonial
Perspective," in *Hermeneutics and Hindu Thought: Toward a Fusion of Horizons*,
ed. Rita D. Sherma and Arvind Sharma (Springer, 2008), 35.

22 Edward Said, *Orientalism* (Knopf Doubleday, 1994), 101.

23 Romila Thapar, *A History of India: Volume 1* (Penguin Books, 1990).

24 Thapar, *A History of India*, 18.

25 Thapar, *A History of India*.

26 Arvind Sharma, "The Hermeneutics of the Word 'Religion' and Its Implications
for the World of Indian Religions," in Sherma and Sharma, *Hermeneutics and
Hindu Thought*, 24.

27 Neha Sahgal et al., "Religion in India: Tolerance and Segregation," Pew Research Center, June 29, 2021, https://www.pewresearch.org/religion/2021/06/29/religion -in-india-tolerance-and-segregation/.

28 Stuart Ray Sarbacker, *Tracing the Path of Yoga* (SUNY Press, 2021).

29 James Mallinson and Mark Singleton, trans., *Roots of Yoga* (Penguin Classics, 2017).

30 Mallinson and Singleton, *Roots of Yoga*, 17.

31 Imma Ramos, *Tantra: Enlightenment to Revolution* (Thames & Hudson, 2020).

32 Mallinson and Singleton, *Roots of Yoga*.

33 Apoorvanand, "Why Is Modi So Scared of History Books?" *Al Jazeera*, April 13, 2023, https://www.aljazeera.com/opinions/2023/4/13/why-is-modi-so-scared-of -history-textbooks.

34 Truschke, *Culture of Encounters*.

35 Rita D. Sherma, introduction to *Hermeneutics and Hindu Thought*, ed. Sherma and Sharma.

36 *Oxford Reference*, "Syncretism," accessed February 26, 2025, https://www .oxfordreference.com/display/10.1093/oi/authority.20110803100547351.

37 Susan Scafidi, *Who Owns Culture? Appropriation and Authenticity in American Law* (Rutgers University Press, 2005), 5.

38 Prachi Patankar, "Ghosts of Yogas Past and Present," *Jadaliyya*, February 26, 2014, https://www.jadaliyya.com/Details/30281.

39 Mia Mingus, "The Four Parts of Accountability & How to Give a Genuine Apology," *Leaving Evidence* (blog), December 18, 2019, https://leavingevidence.wordpress.com /2019/12/18/how-to-give-a-good-apology-part-1-the-four-parts-of-accountability/.

Chapter 3: Sulabha, the Rebellious Philosopher

1 Ruth Vanita, "The Self Is Not Gendered: Sulabha's Debate with King Janaka," *NWSA Journal* 15, no. 2 (2003): 76–93, https://scholarworks.umt.edu/cgi /viewcontent.cgi?article=1001&context=libstudies_pubs.

2 Vanita, "The Self Is Not Gendered."

3 Arti Dhand, *Woman as Fire, Woman as Sage: Sexual Ideology in the Mahābhārata* (SUNY Press, 2009), 30.

4 Dhand, *Woman as Fire*.

5 Dhand, *Woman as Fire*, 36.

6 Uma Chakravarti, *Gendering Caste: Through a Feminist Lens* (Sage Publications, 2018).

7 Michael Witzel, "Female Rishis and Philosophers in the Veda," *Journal of South Asia Women Studies* 11, no. 1 (2009), http://nrs.harvard.edu/urn-3:HUL.InstRepos :9886300.

8 Amara Das Wilhelm, *Tritiya Prakriti: People of the Third Sex: Understanding Homosexuality, Transgender Identity and Intersex Conditions Through Hinduism* (Xlibris US, 2010).

9 Romila Thapar, *A History of India: Volume 1* (Penguin, 1990), 18.

10 Patricia Sauthoff, "Protective Rites in the Netra Tantra" (PhD diss., University of London, 2019), 135, https://eprints.soas.ac.uk/32803/.

11 Poulami Mukherjee, "Theorizing Menstrual Blood: A Tantrik Elixir," 2019, https://www.academia.edu/87790377/Theorizing_Menstrual_Blood_A_Tantrik _Elixir.

12 N. M. Naseera and Moly Kuruvilla, "The Sexual Politics of the Manusmriti: A Critical Analysis with Sexual and Reproductive Health Rights Perspectives," *Journal of International Women's Studies* 23, no. 6 (2022): 3, https://vc.bridgew.edu /cgi/viewcontent.cgi?article=2845&context=jiws.

13 Wendy Doniger and B. K. Smith, trans., *The Laws of Manu* (Penguin Classics, 1991), 208.

14 Chakravarti, *Gendering Caste*.

15 Bhimrao Ambedkar, *Annihilation of Caste: The Annotated Critical Edition* (Verso, 2016).

16 Dhand, *Woman as Fire*, 119.

17 *The Bhagavad Gita: The Transcendental Knowledge* (Srinivas Fine Arts, 2018), 36–38.

18 Chakravarti, *Gendering Caste*, 34.

19 Svatmarama, *The Hatha Yoga Pradipika*, trans. Brian Dana Akers (YogaVidya. com, 2002), 30.

20 Svatmarama, *The Hatha Yoga Pradipika*.

21 Vanita, "The Self Is Not Gendered."

22 Thapar, *A History of India*.

23 Wendy Doniger, *The Hindus: An Alternative History* (Penguin Classics, 2009).

24 M. N. Srinivas, *Caste in Modern India, and Other Essays* (Asia Publishing House, 1957), 48.

25 Doniger and Smith, *The Laws of Manu*, 182.

26 Doniger and Smith, *The Laws of Manu*, 182.

27 Doniger, *The Hindus*.

28 K. Lalita and Susie Tharu, eds., *Women Writing in India: 600 B.C. to the Present. Volume 1: 600 B.C. to the Early Twentieth Century* (Feminist Press, 1991).

29 Lalita and Tharu, *Women Writing in India*, 55.

30 Lalita and Tharu, *Women Writing in India*, 68.

31 Ruth Vanita, *The Dharma of Justice in the Sanskrit Epics: Debates on Gender, Varna, and Species* (Oxford University Press, 2022), 15.

32 Rita D. Sherma, introduction to *Hermeneutics and Hindu Thought: Toward a Fusion of Horizons*, ed. Rita D. Sherma and Arvind Sharma (Springer, 2008).

33 Tracy Pintchman, *The Rise of the Goddess in the Hindu Tradition* (SUNY Press, 1994), 86.

34 Pintchman, *The Rise of the Goddess*, 38.

35 Pupul Jayakar, *The Earthen Drum* (National Museum of Delhi, 1980).

36 Amartya Sen, *The Argumentative Indian* (Picador, 2006).

37 Dhand, *Woman as Fire*, 5.

38 Divya Kandukuri, "The Life and Times of Savitribai Phule," *The Mint Lounge*, December 1, 2019, https://lifestyle.livemint.com/news/talking-point/the-life-and-times-of-savitribai-phule-111642592582316.html.

39 Namrata Namrata, "In Between Honor, Rebellion and Patriarchy: Honor Killings in India," *Global Human Rights Hub fellows blog*, New College of Interdisciplinary Arts and Sciences, Arizona State University, February 9, 2024, https://newcollege.asu.edu/global-human-rights-hub/fellows-program/ghr-fellows-blog/namrata.

40 Meghna Sabharwal, "Rising Gender Inequities in India: The Case of Authoritarian Patriarchy," *Journal of Social Equity and Public Administration* 1, no. 1 (2023): 59–74, https://doi.org/10.24926/jsepa.v1i1.4929.

41 Thenmozhi Soundararajan, *The Trauma of Caste: A Dalit Feminist Meditation on Survivorship, Healing, and Abolition* (North Atlantic Books, 2022), 16, 17.

Chapter 4: The Dance of Radha

1 Namita Gokhale and Malashri Lal, eds., *Finding Radha: The Quest for Love* (Penguin India, 2018).

2 Meghnad Desai, "Radha and the Completion of Krishna," in Gokhale and Lal, *Finding Radha*.

3 Jawhar Sircar, "In Search of the Historical Radha," in Gokhale and Lal, *Finding Radha*, 8.

4 Sircar, "In Search of the Historical Radha."

5 Sircar, "In Search of the Historical Radha."

6 Lavanya Vemsani, "Andal Is our Radha: History and Practice of Hinduism in the Story of Andal in the Telugu, Amuktamalyada of Krishnadevaraya, Vijayanagara Emperor," *International Journal of Dharma and Hindu Studies* 1, no. 2 (2016), https://www.academia.edu/23838998/_Andal_is_our_Radha_History_and_Practice_of_Hinduism_in_the_Story_of_Andal_in_the_Telugu_Amuktamalyada_of_Krishnadevaraya_Vijayanagara_Emperor.

7 K. Lalita and Susie Tharu, eds., *Women Writing in India: 600 B.C. to the Present. Volume 1: 600 B.C. to the Early Twentieth Century* (Feminist Press, 1991), 70.

8   Gokhale and Lal, *Finding Radha.*

9   Barbara Miller, *Gita Govinda of Jayadeva: Love Song of the Dark Lord* (Motilal Banarsidass, 2015).

10 Miller, *Gita Govinda of Jayadeva*, 71.

11 Miller, *Gita Govinda of Jayadeva*, 85.

12 Alka Pande, "Becoming Radha," in Gokhale and Lal, *Finding Radha.*

13 Reba Som, "Radha in Nazrul Geeti," in Gokhale and Lal, *Finding Radha*, 115.

14 VivekaVani, "Krishna – Swami Vivekananda," August 10, 2011, https://vivekavani .com/krishna-swami-vivekananda/. Transcript of a recording of a 1900 speech by Swami Vivekananda.

15 Sircar, "In Search of the Historical Radha."

16 Miller, *Gita Govinda of Jayadeva*, 125.

17 Uma Chakravarti, *Gendering Caste: Through a Feminist Lens* (Sage Publications, 2018), 40.

18 Purushottam Agrawal, *Kabir, Kabir: The Life and Work of the Early Modern Poet-Philosopher* (Westland Non-Fiction, 2024).

19 Agrawal, *Kabir, Kabir*, 45.

20 D. N. Jha, "Brahmanical Intolerance in Early India," *Social Scientist* 44, no. 5/6 (2016): 3–10, www.proquest.com/docview/1809568683?sourcetype=Scholarly Journals.

21 Lalita and Tharu, *Women Writing in India.*

22 Arundhathi Subramaniam, *Wild Women: Seekers, Protagonists and Goddesses in Sacred Indian Poetry* (Ebury Press, 2024), 86.

23 A. K. Ramanujan, *The Collected Essays of A. K. Ramanujan* (Oxford University Press, 1999), 30.

24 Sanjay Kumar et al., "Is Kabir Anti-Women? An Exploratory Study of Kabir's Images Among Kabirpanthi Women," *Journal of Positive School Psychology* 6, no. 3 (2022): 5709, www.journalppw.com/index.php/jpsp/article/view/3258/2118.

25 Anantanand Rambachan, "Caste and Patriarchy: How to Read the 'Ramcharit-manas' of Tulsidas Today," *Scroll*, October 16, 2023, https://scroll.in/article /1055163/caste-and-patriarchy-how-to-read-the-ramcharitmanas-of-tulsidas -today.

Chapter 5: The Naked Truth Tellers

1   Mukunda Rao, *Sky-Clad: The Extraordinary Life and Times of Akka Mahadevi* (Westland, 2018), 19.

2   Rao, *Sky-Clad*, 13.

3   Rao, *Sky-Clad*, 60.

4 Rao, *Sky-Clad*, 60.

5 Rao, *Sky-Clad*, 62.

6 Rao, *Sky-Clad*, 63.

7 M. N. Srinivas, *Caste in Modern India, and Other Essays* (Asia Publishing House, 1957).

8 A. K. Ramanujan, *The Collected Essays of A. K. Ramanujan* (Oxford University Press, 1999), 290.

9 Rao, *Sky-Clad*, 112.

10 Seok Kang, "Disembodiment in Online Social Interaction: Impact of Online Chat on Social Support and Psychosocial Well-Being," *Cyberpsychology, Behavior, and Social Networking* 10, no. 3 (2007): 476, https://doi.org/10.1089/cpb.2006.9929.

Chapter 6: The Song of Piro

1 Anshu Malhotra, *Piro and the Gulabdasis: Gender, Sect and Society in Punjab* (Oxford University Press, 2017), xviii.

2 Neeti Singh, "Peero: Maverick *Bhakta* and First Woman Poet of Punjab," *Indian Literature* 62, no. 4 (306) (2018): 203, https://www.jstor.org/stable/26792168.

3 Singh, "Peero: Maverick *Bhakta*," 204.

4 Malhotra, *Piro and the Gulabdasis*.

5 Arundhathi Subramaniam, *Wild Women: Seekers, Protagonists and Goddesses in Sacred Indian Poetry* (Ebury Press, 2024), 189.

6 Malhotra, *Piro and the Gulabdasis*, 107.

7 Singh, "Peero: Maverick *Bhakta*."

8 Malhotra, *Piro and the Gulabdasis*.

9 Singh, "Peero: Maverick *Bhakta*."

10 Malhotra, *Piro and the Gulabdasis*, 82.

11 Subramaniam, *Wild Women*.

12 Singh, "Peero: Maverick *Bhakta*."

13 Malhotra, *Piro and the Gulabdasis*, 94.

14 Malhotra, *Piro and the Gulabdasis*, 40.

15 Nikky-Guninder Kaur Singh, *Sikhism: An Introduction* (I. B. Tauris, 2011).

16 Gurneet Kaur and Paran Gowda, "Yoga Concept in Sri Guru Granth Sahib Teachings: A Conceptual Frame Development," *Yoga Mimamsa* 53, no. 2 (2021): 129–33, https://doi.org/10.4103/ym.ym_96_21.

17 William Pinch, *Warrior Ascetics and Indian Empires* (Cambridge University Press, 2006), 196.

18 Pluralism Project, "The Khalsa," accessed January 4, 2023, https://pluralism.org
   /the-khalsa.

19 Malhotra, *Piro and the Gulabdasis.*

20 Malhotra, *Piro and the Gulabdasis.*

21 Anita M. Leopold and Jeppe Sinding Jensen, eds., *Syncretism in Religion: A
   Reader* (Routledge, 2014).

22 "Advayataraka Upanishad," VyasaOnline.com, accessed February 26, 2024, https://
   www.vyasaonline.com/advayataraka-upanishad.

23 Matthew Remski, "Yoga's Culture of Sexual Abuse: Nine Women Tell Their Stories," *The Walrus*, April 25, 2018, https://thewalrus.ca/yogas-culture-of-sexual
   -abuse-nine-women-tell-their-stories/.

24 Jivana Heyman, *Yoga Revolution: Building a Practice of Courage and Compassion*
   (Shambala, 2021), 45–49.

Conclusion: Embodied Resistance

1 Laura Silver and Janell Fetterolf, "Who Likes Authoritarianism, and How Do They
   Want to Change Their Government?" Pew Research Center, February 28, 2024,
   https://www.pewresearch.org/short-reads/2024/02/28/who-likes-authoritarianism
   -and-how-do-they-want-to-change-their-government/.

2 Shambuka, "Neoliberalizing Racial Justice: Caste, Race, and Diaspora Hindutva
   Democrats," *Peace & Change* 46, no. 4 (2021): 384–402, https://doi.org/10.1111
   /pech.12492.

3 Political Research Associates and Savera: United Against Supremacy, *HAF Way to
   Supremacy: How the Hindu American Foundation Rebrands Bigotry as Minority
   Rights*, 2024, https://www.wearesavera.org/wp-content/uploads/2024/10
   /HAFWaytoSupremacy.pdf.

4 Maari Zwick-Maitreyi et al., *Caste in the United States: A Survey of Caste Among
   South Asian Americans* (Equality Labs, 2018), https://equalitylabs.wpengine.com
   /wp-content/uploads/2023/10/Caste_in_the_United_States_Report2018.pdf.

5 "Love, Power and Liberation," panel discussion with Angela Davis and Lama Rod
   Owens, fundraiser to support East Bay Meditation Center, Oakland, CA, November 8, 2024.

Bibliography

Agrawal, Purushottam. *Kabir, Kabir: The Life and Work of the Early Modern Poet-Philosopher.* Westland Non-Fiction, 2024.

Ambedkar, Bhimrao. *Annihilation of Caste: The Annotated Critical Edition.* Verso, 2016.

Amnesty International. "India: Authorities Must End Repression of Dissent in Jammu and Kashmir." Amnesty International, September 18, 2024. https://www.amnesty.org/en/latest/news/2024/09/india-authorities-must-end-repression-of-dissent-in-jammu-and-kashmir/.

Anjum, Tanvir. "The Emergence of Muslim Rule in India: Some Historical Disconnects and Missing Links." *Islamic Studies* 46, no. 2 (2007): 217–40. https://www.jstor.org/stable/20839068.

Apoorvanand. "Why Is Modi So Scared of History Books?" *Al Jazeera*, April 13, 2023. https://www.aljazeera.com/opinions/2023/4/13/why-is-modi-so-scared-of-history-textbooks.

Barua, Ankur, and Vishal Vasanthakumar. "Renaming Caste, Retaining Privilege." *The India Forum*, June 15, 2024. https://www.theindiaforum.in/caste/renaming-caste-retaining-privilege

The Bhagavad Gita: The Transcendental Knowledge. Srinivas Fine Arts, 2018.

Biswas, Soutik. "Oppenheimer: How He Was Influenced by the Bhagavad Gita." *BBC*, July 24, 2023. https://www.bbc.com/news/world-asia-india-66288900.

Bouillier, Veronique. "Aurangzeb and the Nāth Yogīs." *Journal of the Royal Asiatic Society* 28, no. 3 (2018): 525–35. https://doi.org/10.1017/S1356186318000081.

Calamur, Krishnadev. "Calif. Judge Rules Yoga in Public Schools Not Religious." *NPR*, July 1, 2013. https://www.npr.org/sections/thetwo-way/2013/07/01/197712791/calif-judge-rules-yoga-in-public-schools-not-religious.

Chakravarti, Uma. *Gendering Caste: Through a Feminist Lens.* Sage Publications, 2018.

Das, Gurcharan. *The Difficulty of Being Good: On the Subtle Art of Dharma.* Oxford University Press, 2010.

Debroy, Bibek. *Valmiki Ramayana.* India Penguin Classics, 2017.

Desai, Meghnad. "Radha and the Completion of Krishna." In Gokhale and Lal, *Finding Radha*.

Dhand, Arti. *Woman as Fire, Woman as Sage: Sexual Ideology in the Mahābhārata*. SUNY Press, 2008.

Doniger, Wendy. *The Hindus: An Alternative History*. Penguin Classics, 2009.

Doniger, Wendy, and B. K. Smith, trans. *The Laws of Manu*. Penguin Classics, 1991.

Eraly, Abraham. *Gem in the Lotus: The Seeding of Indian Civilisation*. Penguin Books India, 2000.

Ernst, Carl. *Refractions of Islam in India: Situating Sufism and Yoga*. Sage Publications, 2016.

Gokhale, Namita, and Malashri Lal, eds. *Finding Radha: The Quest for Love*. Penguin India, 2018.

Hebbar, Nistula. "Rig Veda Golden Age for Women's Rights: Sangh History Body." *The Hindu*, September 20, 2015. https://www.thehindu.com/news/national/rig -veda-golden-age-for-womens-rights-sangh-history-body/article7669178.ece.

Heyman, Jivana. *Yoga Revolution: Building a Practice of Courage and Compassion*. Shambala, 2021, 45–49.

Hiltebeitel, Alf. *The Cult of Draupadi: Mythologies From Gingee to Kurukshetra*. Vol 1. University of Chicago Press, 1991.

HT Correspondent. "Ramdev Offers to 'Cure Homosexuals' at His Haridwar Ashram." *Hindustan Times*, December 11, 2013. https://www.hindustantimes. com/india/ramdev-offers-to-cure-homosexuals-at-his-haridwar-ashram/story -UtnktIHM8qAdT5NKbG7QsO.html.

Jain, Andrea R. *Peace Love Yoga: The Politics of Global Spirituality*. Oxford Academic, 2020.

Jayakar, Pupul. *The Earthen Drum*. National Museum of Delhi, 1980.

Jha, D. N. "Brahmanical Intolerance in Early India." *Social Scientist* 44, no. 5/6 (2016): 3–10. www.proquest.com/docview/1809568683?sourcetype=ScholarlyJournals.

Jha, D. N. *The Myth of the Holy Cow*. Verso, 2002.

Joseph, Tony. *Early Indians: The Story of Our Ancestors and Where We Came From*. Juggernaut, 2018.

Kandukuri, Divya. "The Life and Times of Savitribai Phule." *The Mint Lounge*, December 1, 2019. https://lifestyle.livemint.com/news/talking-point/the-life-and -times-of-savitribai-phule-111642592582316.html.

Kang, Seok. "Disembodiment in Online Social Interaction: Impact of Online Chat on Social Support and Psychosocial Well-Being." *Cyberpsychology, Behavior, and Social Networking* 10, no. 3 (2007): 475–77. https://doi.org/10.1089/cpb .2006.9929.

Katz, Tristan (@tristankatzcreative). "Additionally, I wonder if folks consider non-binary and genderfluid individuals when using womxn and women+." Instagram, November 18, 2024. https://www.instagram.com/p/DChRIUevVly/?img_index =6&igsh=MzRlODBiNWFlZA==.

Kaur, Gurneet, and Paran Gowda. "Yoga Concept in Sri Guru Granth Sahib Teachings: A Conceptual Frame Development." *Yoga Mimamsa* 53, no. 2 (2021): 129–33. https://doi.org/10.4103/ym.ym_96_21.

Kinsley, David. *Hindu Goddesses: Visions of the Divine Feminine in the Hindu Religious Traditions*. University of California Press, 1988.

Kumar, Sanjay, Ajit Mishra, and Veeru Rajbhar. "Is Kabir Anti-Women? An Exploratory Study of Kabir's Images Among Kabirpanthi Women." *Journal of Positive School Psychology* 6, no. 3 (2022): 5709–18. www.journalppw.com/index.php /jpsp/article/view/3258/2118.

Lalita, K., and Susie Tharu, eds. *Women Writing in India: 600 B.C. to the Present. Volume 1: 600 B.C. to the Early Twentieth Century*. Feminist Press, 1991.

Leopold, Anita M., and Jeppe Sinding Jensen, eds. *Syncretism in Religion: A Reader*. Routledge, 2014.

Lerner, Gerda. *Living with History/Making Social Change*. University of North Carolina Press, 2009.

Lorenzen, David. "Who Invented Hinduism?" *Comparative Studies in Society and History* 41, no. 4 (1999): 630–59. https://doi.org/10.1017/S0010417599003084.

Mahalaksmi, R. "Sanatana Dharma's Historical Roots Reveal a Complex Journey." *Frontline*, October 5, 2023. https://frontline.thehindu.com/the-nation/essay -r-mahalakshmi-on-sanatana-dharma-historical-interpretations-contemporary -concerns-roots-reveal-a-complex-journey/article67326266.ece.

Malhotra, Anshu. *Piro and the Gulabdasis: Gender, Sect and Society in Punjab*. Oxford University Press, 2017.

Mallinson, James, and Mark Singleton, trans. *Roots of Yoga*. Penguin Classics, 2017.

Miller, Barbara. *Gita Govinda of Jayadeva: Love Song of the Dark Lord*. Motilal Banarsidass, 2015.

Mingus, Mia. "The Four Parts of Accountability & How to Give a Genuine Apology." *Leaving Evidence* (blog), December 18, 2019. https://leavingevidence.wordpress.com /2019/12/18/how-to-give-a-good-apology-part-1-the-four-parts-of-accountability/.

Modi, Narendra. "Statement by H. E. Narendra Modi, Prime Minister of India." General Debate of the 69th Session of the United Nations General Assembly. September 27, 2014. https://www.un.org/en/ga/69/meetings/gadebate/pdf/IN_en.pdf.

Mogul, Rhea. "Modi's Muslim Remarks Spark 'Hate Speech' Accusations as India's Mammoth Election Deepens Divides." *CNN*, April 22, 2024. https://www.cnn

.com/2024/04/22/asia/india-modi-muslim-hate-speech-allegations-intl-hnk
/index.html.

Mukherjee, Poulami. "Theorizing Menstrual Blood: A Tantrik Elixir." 2019. https://
www.academia.edu/87790377/Theorizing_Menstrual_Blood_A_Tantrik_Elixir.

Namrata, Namrata. "In Between Honor, Rebellion and Patriarchy: Honor Killings in
India." *Global Human Rights Hub fellows blog*, New College of Interdisciplinary
Arts and Sciences, Arizona State University, February 9, 2024. https://newcollege
.asu.edu/global-human-rights-hub/fellows-program/ghr-fellows-blog/namrata.

Naseera, N. M., and Moly Kuruvilla. "The Sexual Politics of the Manusmriti: A Critical Analysis with Sexual and Reproductive Health Rights Perspectives." *Journal of
International Women's Studies* 23, no. 6 (2022): 3. https://vc.bridgew.edu/cgi
/viewcontent.cgi?article=2845&context=jiws.

Omvedt, Gail. *Understanding Caste: From Buddha to Ambedkar and Beyond*. Orient
Black Swan, 2012.

Pande, Alka. "Becoming Radha." In Gokhale and Lal, *Finding Radha*.

Pande, Mrinal. "Gendered Analysis of Hindutva Imaginaries: Manipulation of Symbols for Ethnonationalist Projects." *Journal of Modern European History* 20, no. 3
(2022): 407–22. https://doi.org/10.1177/16118944221110725.

Patankar, Prachi. "Ghosts of Yogas Past and Present." *Jadaliyya*, February 26, 2014.
https://www.jadaliyya.com/Details/30281.

Pillai, Manu. "A Mosque Celebrating a Hindu King." *Manu S. Pillai* (blog), November 14, 2019. https://manuspillai.com/2019/11/14/a-mosque-celebrating-a-hindu
-king-16-november-2019/.

Pinch, William. *Warrior Ascetics and Indian Empires*. Cambridge University Press, 2006.

Pintchman, Tracy. *The Rise of the Goddess in the Hindu Tradition*. SUNY Press, 1994.

Pluralism Project. "The Khalsa." Pluralism Project, Harvard University. Accessed January 4, 2023. https://pluralism.org/the-khalsa.

Political Research Associates and Savera: United Against Supremacy. *HAF Way to
Supremacy: How the Hindu American Foundation Rebrands Bigotry as Minority
Rights*. Political Research Associates, 2024. https://www.wearesavera.org/wp
-content/uploads/2024/10/HAFWaytoSupremacy.pdf.

Ramanujan, A. K. *The Collected Essays of A. K. Ramanujan*. Oxford University Press,
1999.

Rambachan, Anantanand. "Caste and Patriarchy: How to Read the Ramcharitmanas
of Tulsidas Today." *Scroll*, October 16, 2023. https://scroll.in/article/1055163
/caste-and-patriarchy-how-to-read-the-ramcharitmanas-of-tulsidas-today.

Ramos, Imma. *Tantra: Enlightenment to Revolution*. Thames & Hudson, 2020.

Rao, Mukunda. *Sky-Clad: The Extraordinary Life and Times of Akka Mahadevi*. Westland, 2018.

Ray, Sunanda K. Datta. "Secularism Is the Core Safeguard India Needs." *Deccan Chronicle*, December 31, 2018. https://www.deccanchronicle.com/opinion /columnists/010119/secularism-is-the-core-safeguard-india-needs.html.

Remski, Matthew. "Yoga's Culture of Sexual Abuse: Nine Women Tell Their Stories." *The Walrus*, April 25, 2018. https://thewalrus.ca/yogas-culture-of-sexual-abuse -nine-women-tell-their-stories/.

Sabharwal, Meghna. "Rising Gender Inequities in India: The Case of Authoritarian Patriarchy." *Journal of Social Equity and Public Administration* 1, no. 1 (2023): 59–74. https://doi.org/10.24926/jsepa.v1i1.4929.

Sahgal, Neha, Jonathan Evans, Ariana Monique Salazar, Kelsey Jo Starr, and Manolo Corichi. "Religion in India: Tolerance and Segregation." Pew Research Center, June 29, 2021. https://www.pewresearch.org/religion/2021/06/29/religion -in-india-tolerance-and-segregation/.

Said, Edward. *Orientalism*. Knopf Doubleday, 1994.

Sarbacker, Stuart Ray. *Tracing the Path of Yoga*. SUNY Press, 2021.

Sauthoff, Patricia. "Protective Rites in the Netra Tantra" (PhD diss., University of London, 2019). https://eprints.soas.ac.uk/32803/.

Scafidi, Susan. *Who Owns Culture? Appropriation and Authenticity in American Law*. Rutgers University Press, 2005.

Sen, Amartya. *The Argumentative Indian*. Picador, 2006.

Shambuka. "Neoliberalizing Racial Justice: Caste, Race, and Diaspora Hindutva Democrats." *Peace & Change* 46, no. 4 (2021): 384–402. https://doi.org/10.1111 /pech.12492.

Sharma, Arvind. "The Hermeneutics of the Word 'Religion' and Its Implications for the World of Indian Religions." In *Hermeneutics and Hindu Thought: Toward a Fusion of Horizons*, edited by Rita D. Sherma and Arvind Sharma, 19–32. Springer, 2008.

Sharma, Rakhi (@_spiritual_therapy). "Hindu push-ups For Beginners." https:// www.instagram.com/reel/C8wryNOPnlN/?igsh=NTc4MTIwNjQ2YQ==.

Sherma, Rita D. Introduction to *Hermeneutics and Hindu Thought: Toward a Fusion of Horizons*. Edited by Rita D. Sherma and Arvind Sharma, 1–18. Springer, 2008.

Silver, Laura, and Janell Fetterolf. "Who Likes Authoritarianism, and How Do They Want to Change Their Government?" Pew Research Center, February 28, 2024. https://www.pewresearch.org/short-reads/2024/02/28/who-likes-authoritarianism -and-how-do-they-want-to-change-their-government/.

Singh, Neeti. "Peero: Maverick *Bhakta* and First Woman Poet of Punjab." *Indian Literature* 62, no. 4 (306) (2018): 201–13. https://www.jstor.org/stable/26792168.

Singh, Nikky-Guninder Kaur. *Sikhism: An Introduction*. I. B. Tauris, 2011.

Sircar, Jawhar. "In Search of the Historical Radha." In Gokhale and Lal, *Finding Radha*.

Som, Reba. "Radha in Nazrul Geeti." In Gokhale and Lal, *Finding Radha*.

Sood, Sheena. "Om-Washing: Why Modi's Yoga Day Pose Is Deceptive." *Al Jazeera*, June 22, 2023. https://www.aljazeera.com/opinions/2023/6/22/om-washing -modis-yoga-day-pose-of-deception.

Soundararajan, Thenmozhi. *The Trauma of Caste: A Dalit Feminist Meditation on Survivorship, Healing, and Abolition*. North Atlantic Books, 2022.

Southworth, Franklin, and David McAlpin. "30 South Asia: Dravidian Linguistic History." *The Encyclopedia of Global Human Migration*, February 4, 2013. https:// doi.org/10.1002/9781444351071.wbeghm830.

Srinivas, M. N. *Caste in Modern India, and Other Essays*. Asia Publishing House, 1957.

Subramaniam, Arundhathi. *Wild Women: Seekers, Protagonists and Goddesses in Sacred Indian Poetry*. Ebury Press, 2024.

Sugirtharajah, Sharada. "Max Mueller and Textual Management: A Postcolonial Perspective." In *Hermeneutics and Hindu Thought: Toward a Fusion of Horizons*, edited by Rita D. Sherma and Arvind Sharma, 33–44. Springer, 2008.

Svatmarama. *The Hatha Yoga Pradipika*. Translated by Brian Dana Akers. YogaVidya .com, 2002.

Thapar, Romila. *The Future in the Past: Essays and Reflections*. Aleph Book Company, 2023.

Thapar, Romila. *A History of India: Volume 1*. Penguin, 1990.

Tharuvana, Azeez. *Living Ramayanas: Exploring the Plurality of the Epic in Wayanad and the World*. Eka, 2021.

Truschke, Audrey. *Culture of Encounters: Sanskrit at the Mughal Court*. Penguin Random House India, 2017.

Udupa, Deeksha, and Raqib Hameed Naik. "The Hindu Nationalist Campaign to Promote Yoga." *The Nation*, April 6, 2023. https://www.thenation.com/article /culture/yogathon-hindu-nationalism/.

Vanita, Ruth. *The Dharma of Justice in the Sanskrit Epics: Debates on Gender, Varna, and Species*. Oxford University Press, 2022.

Vanita, Ruth. "The Self Is Not Gendered: Sulabha's Debate with King Janaka." *NWSA Journal* 15, no. 2 (2003): 76–93. https://scholarworks.umt.edu /cgi/viewcontent.cgi?article=1001&context=libstudies_pubs.

Vásquez, Ian, Fred McMahon, Ryan Murphy, and Guillermina Sutter Schneider. *The Human Freedom Index 2023: A Global Measurement of Personal, Civic, and Economic Freedom*. Cato Institute and Fraser Institute, 2023. https://www.cato.org /human-freedom-index/2023.

Vemsani, Lavanya. "Andal Is our Radha: History and Practice of Hinduism in the Story of Andal in the Telugu, Amuktamalyada of Krishnadevaraya, Vijayanagara Emperor." *International Journal of Dharma and Hindu Studies* 1, no. 2 (2016). https://www.academia.edu/23838998/_Andal_is_our_Radha _History_and_Practice_of_Hinduism_in_the_Story_of_Andal_in_the_Telugu _Amuktamalyada_of_Krishnadevaraya_Vijayanagara_Emperor.

VivekaVani. "Krishna – Swami Vivekananda." August 10, 2011. https://vivekavani .com/krishna-swami-vivekananda/.

Waikar, Prashant. "Reading Islamophobia in Hindutva: An Analysis of Narendra Modi's Political Discourse." *Islamophobia Studies Journal* 4, no. 2 (2018): 161–80. https://doi.org/10.13169/islastudj.4.2.0161.

Wilhelm, Amara Das. *Tritiya Prakriti: People of the Third Sex: Understanding Homosexuality, Transgender Identity and Intersex Conditions Through Hinduism*. Xlibris US, 2010.

Witzel, Michael. "Female Rishis and Philosophers in the Veda." *Journal of South Asia Women Studies* 11, no. 1 (2009). http://nrs.harvard.edu/urn-3:HUL.InstRepos :9886300.

Zwick-Maitreyi, Maari, Thenmozhi Soundararajan, Natasha Dar, Ralph F. Bheel, and Prathap Balakrishnan. *Caste in the United States: A Survey of Caste Among South Asian Americans*. Equality Labs, 2018. https://equalitylabs.wpengine.com /wp-content/uploads/2023/10/Caste_in_the_United_States_Report2018.pdf.

Index

A

abhinaya, 11
abhyasa, 168
Aditi, 31, 88
Adivasis, 37
Advaita Vedanta, 33, 69
Agni, 30, 88, 97
Alexander the Great, 65
Ambedkar, Bhimrao, 12, 38, 52
Amritasiddhi, 68
Ananda, 98
Ananta asana, 48
Andal, 115
animal sacrifices, Vedic pastoralists, 31–33
Annihilation of Caste (Ambedkar), 38
Anyaradhita, 115
apology, 77
appropriation and appreciation of yoga, 74–77, 170
    Radha, 132–133
Aranyakas, 41
archetypes
    influence of, 104–105
    Vedic Brahmanism, 93
Arjuna, 13, 85, 95
    gender fluidity, 101
    Kali Yuga, 92
    Krishna, 91
artha, 84
asanas
    named after deities, 48
    need for embodiment practices, 148
    Sanskrit, 106
    Upanishadic and Patanjala yoga, 68
ascetic, 84–86
ashramas, 50, 83
    vanaprastha ashrama, 86

astikas and nastikas, 51
astrology, 88
Asvins, 32
Atharva Veda, 32, 41
Atma, 70, 99, 109
    gender, 82
Aurangzeb, 60, 160–161
Austroasiatic languages, 26
authoritarian regimes, 168
avarnas, 57
    British colonization, 62–63
    preservation of class and caste in Manu
        Smriti, 96–97
avidya, 167
Awadhi, 130
ayurveda, purity and pollution, 108

B

Baba Ramdev, 5
Bahadur, Guru Tegh, 161
Bahr-al-Hayat, 60
Bahujan, 37
balakrishna, 121
Balarama, 122
Basavanna, 140–146
Beef, Vedic pastoralists, 31–33
Bhagavad Gita, 1, 8, 11–12, 14, 25, 54
    Arjuna, 95
    composition of, 68
    gender fluidity, 99
    horse-chariot/ox-cart metaphor, 64, 66
    Krishna, 118, 124
    Krishna and Arjuna, 85
    lack of word *Hindu*, 50
    Mahabharata, 17
    portrayal of women, 102
    preference over oral traditions, 147

Bhagavad Gita (*continued*)
    references to yoga, 67–68
    shared feature with *Gita Govinda*, 131
    Swami Vivekananda, 122
Bhagavat Purana, 115, 123
    Krishna, 118
    preference over oral traditions, 147
bhakti, 11, 52, 68, 124–131. *See also* Radha
    Akka Mahadevi. *See* Mahadevi, Akka
    Basavanna, 143–146
    Bhakti saints, 128
    bridal mysticism, 138–139
    caste-privileged Bhakti poets, 129–131
    castes, 127–130
    challenge to Brahmanical patriarchy, 98, 109
    challenge to gender, 145
    conflict among Bhakti factions, 127
    confronting patriarchal norms, 130
    Kabir, 126–127
    Krishna, 115, 119–120
    marga, 68, 71, 124, 156
    nine forms of, 125
    Piro and Gulabdas, 154, 157
    poetry about women's labor and drudgery,
        128–129
    Radha, 112, 114, 119, 125–126
    rasa as resistance, 131–132
    supporters of Prime Minister Narendra
        Modi, 131
    village deities, 124
    viveka, 133–134
    yoga, 124, 134
Bhakti movement, 9, 45, 59–60, 98, 115, 128
    class and caste, 130
Bhakti poetry, 57–58, 120, 125
    surrender to guru, 157
Bharatiya Janata Party, 168
Bhimbekta cave paintings, 87
Bhishma, 101
Brahma Vaivarta, 116
Brahman, 70
Brahmanas, 41
Brahmanism, ix–x, 12, 24
    acknowledgement of Brahmanization in
        yoga, 170
    archetypes in Vedic Brahmanism, 93
    Brahmanical orthodoxy/Vedic Brahmanism, 9
    establishment of, 37–40
    expanding inquiries of Brahmanical
        patriarchy in yoga history, 108–109
    Kalabhras dynasty, 143
    origin of, 35–36

Radha: Brahmanism, appropriation, and
    sanitization, 132–133
Sanskrit as medium for, 94–98
sex and control, 90–91
Tantra, 89–90
Vedic literature, 40–45
Brahmins, 35
    conflicts with Buddhists, 39
    dharma for Brahmin men, 88–89
    foundational myth of Brahmin class, 34
    women, 87
Braj, 159
breath, ix
bridal mysticism, 138–139
Brihannala, 101
British
    colonization, 61–63
    recognition of castes, 94
    recognition of Hindus, 61
    translation of Sanskrit texts, 62, 94
Buddha, 65
    foster mother, Mahapajapathi Gotami, 98
    and women, 97–98
Buddhism/Buddhists, 24, 56
    conflicts with Brahmins, 39
    gurus, 164
    ideals for society and role state, 39–40
    Kalabhras dynasty, 143
    monks, 167–168
    nastikas, 51
    patriarchy, 98
    schools, 57
    Therigatha or Songs of the Buddhist Nuns,
        97–98
bulls, Vedic pastoralists, 31–33
burning of Manu Smriti, 94

C

capitalism
    assignment of value, 132
    neoliberal spiritual capitalism, 4–5, 170
caste, x
    1872 and 1881 censuses, 94
    abolitionists, 12
    in Bhagavad Gita, 12
    bhakti, 127–130
    diaspora, 168
    Ekalavya and Dronacharya, 97
    emergence of, 52
    feminist resistance, 105
    genesis of, 34
    history, 34–36

jaatis, 36–37
Kalabhras dynasty, 143
karma, 42
Manu Smriti, 96–97
oppression, 13, 52–53
patriarchy as part of caste system, 86–90
prevalence among religions of South Asia, 60
prohibition of intermarriage, 43
recognition by British, 94
Sanskritization, 96
sex and control, 90–91
temples, 127–128
untouchability, 38
cave paintings at Bhimbekta, 87
Chakravarti, Uma, 12, 14
Chandala, 39
Chandogya Upanishad, 121
changed behavior, 77
chanti lingam, 102
Charvakas, 9
Chatterji, Angana, 7
Chaturanga, 48
Chausath Yogini temple, 104
Chennamallikarjuna, 137–139, 141–142
Cheraman Jumma Masjid mosque, 59
child marriage, 90
Chowdhury, Bikram, 164
cisgender in Vedic literature, 88
classes
Bhakti movement, 130
history, 34–36
Manu Smriti, 96–97
sexual intermingling (varnasamkara), 91–92
cocreating welcoming yoga spaces, 170
commentaries on texts, 69
consciousness, Upanishads, 70
control and sex, 90–94
cows, Vedic pastoralists, 31–33
cultural appropriation of yoga, 74–77
curry, Hinduism analogy, 48–50

D
Dalits, 37
barring from Puranic temples, 127–128
crimes against, 106
Dara Shikoh, 60
Dasa, 35
women, 91
Dasas, 34
Dattatreyayogasastra, 69
Davis, Angela, 171

debates as resistance, 103–106
Ded, Lal, 147
deities. *See* gods and goddesses
Desikachar, 69
devadasis, 119
Devas, conflicts with Rakshasas, 37
Devi, 11, 51
asana, 48
Puranas, 17
yoga studios, 48
Devi Bhagavata, 116
Devi, Ila, 123
Devi, Indra, 69, 104
dhamma, 39
Dhand, Arti, 14, 84
dharma, 1, 13, 41, 42, 50, 53–56
Brahmin men, 88–89
four purusharthas, 84
law texts, 42–43
Manu Smriti definition of whom dharma applies, 50
nivritti dharma, 84–86, 92, 101
pravritti dharma, 84–86, 92, 101
reinforcement through storytelling, 17
sanatan, 24
stri dharma, 90
women, 40
Dharmashastras, 41, 54
Manava Dharmashastra. *See* Manava Dharmashastra (aka Manu Smriti)
pravritti dharma, 85
self-referential, 43
diaspora, 168
diet, purity and pollution, 108
Digambaras monks, 145–146
Din-Ilahi, 161
discernment (viveka), 133–134
disembodiment, 19
dissonance, xi, 14
Divyadana, 127
Diwali, observance at yoga studios, 48
dogmatism, x
Draupadi, 18, 101
Dravidian languages, 29
Dronacharya, 97
dukka, 70–71, 76
Dyaus, 31

E
The Earthen Drum (Jayakar), 23
East India Company, 94
Ekalavya, 11, 13, 97

Eka-Sringi, 23
Eknath, 130
embodied action, 171–172
embodied resistance, 18–19
    sacred resilience, 18–19
embodiment, 148
    nakedness. *See* nakedness
    radical, 148–149
Emperor Akbar, 59
Equality Labs, 38

F

feminist resistance to caste, 105
festival celebrations in yoga studios, 48
fetus in womb, 83
four levels of analysis of myth, 13
four purusharthas, 84

G

Gandhari, 35
Ganesha
    depiction in yoga studios, 48
    Puranas, 17
Gargi, 81, 87, 104, 108
Gatha Saptasati, 114, 115
Gautam Buddha, 38, 65
gender, 82–83
    archetypes in Vedic Brahmanism, 93
    Atma, 82
    bhakti challenge to gender, 145
    development of fetus in womb, 83
    diverse gender identities in Vedic literature, 88
    men and women in Manava Dharmashastra, 88–89
    pums (man) prakriti, 88
    stri (woman) prakriti, 88
    trittiya prakriti, 88
    Sulabha, 82–83
    Vedic astrology, 88
gender fluidity, 82, 99–103
Gherandasamhita, 69
Gita, 66
    Bhagavad Gita. *See* Bhagavad Gita
    Kali Yuga, 92
    varnasamkara, 91–92
    yoga teacher training, 47
Gita Govinda, 14, 116–119, 123–124
    shared features with Bhagavad Gita, 131
The God of Small Things (Roy), 79
goddesses, 87–88. *See also* gods and goddesses
    bhakti. *See* bhakti
    Chausath Yogini temple, 104

goddess worship, 86
    Hindu theism, 51–52
    Lakshmi, 113
    Saraswati, 96, 113
    Vak, 100
    in Vedas, 30–31
godhadi, 3
gods and goddesses, 50. *See also* goddesses
    bhakti. *See* bhakti
    Hindu theism, 51–52
    homosexual relationships, 88
    in Vedas, 30–31, 97
    village deities, 124
Gondi, 29
Gopatha Brahmana, 32
Gotami, Mahapajapathi, 98
government
    authoritarian regimes, 168
    India prime minister Narendra Modi, 5–6, 131
    Public Safety Act and the Unlawful Activities Prevention Act, 6–7
    section 375 of the Indian Penal Code, 105
grama devatas, 124
Great Goddess, 18
Gulabdas, 158–162, 169
    bhakti of Piro, 154, 157
    burial with Piro, 157, 162
    intimate relationships with women, 161
    "jog and bhog", 161
    meeting Piro, 153–154
    Nath yogis, 160
    rejection of varna-ashrama-dharma, 159
    sant, 161, 162
    soham, 159
    syncretism, 162
Gulabdasis, 153
gurus, 163–166
    Gulabdas. *See* Gulabdas
    sexual misconduct accusations, 164–165
    Sikhs/Sikhism, 159–160
    surrender to, 157

H

Hala, 114
Hanuman asana, 48
Harappans, 27–30, 32
    languages, 95
Hare Krishna, 120
Hari, 122
Harivamsa, 122
hatha yoga, 25, 68

convergence with Patanjali's yoga, 69
women, 92–93, 102
Hatha Yoga Pradipika (Svatmarama), 12, 69, 92–93, 102
   expanding inquiries of Brahmanical patriarchy, 109
   preference over oral traditions, 147
   yoga teacher training, 47
Hedgewar, K. B., 6
heterodoxy, 9–10, 24
   bhakti, 130
   nastikas, 51
himsa, 32
Hindu American Foundation, 8
Hindu, and yoga, 47–53
   definition of yoga, 64–70
   dharma, 53–56
   genesis of "Hindu" label, 56–64
   yoga teacher training and yoga studios, 47–48
Hinduism
   bhakti, 52
   caste, 52, 53
   curry analogy, 49–50
   definition of, 52
   geopolitical identification, 49–50
   genesis as an -ism, 56–64
   Islam's connection to India, 58, 59, 60, 61
   myth of Hindu society, 52
   origin of word *Hindu*, 49
   religious nationalism. *See* Hindutva
   theism, 51, 52
Hinduism, origin of
   archaeological history, 25–27
   emergence of jaati, 34–40
   Harappans, 27–30
   Vedic literature and Brahmanism, 40–45
   Vedic pastoralists, 30–33
Hindus
   Indigeneity, 74
   Lal Ded, 147
   pluralism, 71–74
   polarities between Hindus and Muslims, 61–62
Hindutva, 5–11, 23, 24, 134
   heterodoxy, 9–10
   Prime Minister Narendra Modi, 5–6, 131
   Take Back Yoga campaign, 8
   United States, 168
   Vinayak Damodar Savarkar, 94
history, 1–5
   British colonizers' recognition of Hindus, 61
   castes and classes, 34–36

conveyed through storytelling, 16–18
emergence of jaati, 34–40
establishment of Brahmanism, 37–40
Harappans, 27–30
heterodoxy, 9–10
Hinduism, 56–64
Hindutva, 5–11
Homo sapiens, 25–26
India, 25–27. *See also* India history
Islam's connection to India, 58–61
languages, 24, 26, 29–30
neoliberal spiritual capitalism, 4–5
paintings, 72
reexamining yoga history, 4–5
resistance against oppression, 3–4
Sanskrit, 95
South Asia, 26–27
Vedic Age, 35
Vedic literature and Brahmanism, 40–45
Vedic pastoralists, 30–33
Vedic people (Indo-Aryans), 26–27
women in yoga, 104
The History of British India (Mill), 61–62
holding multiplicities, 109
Holi, observance by yoga studios, 48
Homo sapiens, 25–26
homosexual relationships among deities, 88
honor killings, 105–106
hot yoga, 164
householder (pravritti dharma), 84–86, 92, 101
   mutual dependence, 168
hybridization, 162–163

I

Ik Sau Sath Kafian (Piro), 153–156
India
   connection to Islam, 58–61
   Hindutva. *See* Hindutva
   history. *See* India history
   Prime Minister Narendra Modi, 5–6, 131
   Public Safety Act and the Unlawful Activities Prevention Act, 6–7
   religious nationalism. *See* Hindutva, 7
India history, 25–27
   archaeology, 25–27
   emergence of jaati, 34–40
   establishment of Brahmanism, 37–40
   Harappans, 27–30
   Indo-Aryans (Vedic people), 26–27
   Vedic literature and Brahmanism, 40–45
   Vedic pastoralists, 30–33
Indigeneity, 24, 74

Indo-Aryans (Vedic people), 26–27
Indra, 32, 97
Indrani, 87
Indus Valley Civilization, 27
Integral Yoga, 164
integrating and synthesize new learnings, 171
interconnectedness, 167
interdependence among all of creation, 167
International Day of Yoga, 6
International Society for Krishna Consciousness
    (ISKCON/Hare Krishna), 120
intersectional feminism, 105
intersex, 88
intertextuality, 41, 43
Ishwara, 101
ISKCON (International Society for Krishna
    Consciousness), 120
Islam. *See also* Muslims
    connection to India, 58–61
    Din-Ilahi, 161
    Indigeneity, 74
    pluralism, 71–74
    synergies between Islam and yoga, 72
Islam, Kazi Nazrul, 120
itihasa, 16
Iyengar, B. K. S., 8, 69

J

jaatis, 36–37
    emergence of jaati, 34–40
    prohibition of intermarriage, 43
Jagannatha, 118, 132
Jains/Jainism, 24, 38, 56
    Digambaras monks, 145, 146
    gurus, 164
    Kalabhras dynasty, 143
    nastikas, 51
    patriarchy, 98
    Radha in drama and literature, 115
    references to yoga, 66
    schools, 57
    Shvetambara monks, 146
Jalauka, 127
Janabai, 128–130, 169
Janaka, 93
    Sulabha, 80–83
Jayadeva, 116–118, 131. *See also Gita Govinda*
Jayakar, Pupul, 23
Jha, D. N., 33
jivanmrit, 126
"jog and bhog", *161*

Jois, Pattabhi, 8, 69, 164
Jones, William, 94

K

Kabir, 58, 126–127, 130, 132, 146, 156, 169
kaivalya, 70
Kalabhras dynasty, 143
Kali Yuga, 92
Kalyana, 140
kama, 84
Kanaka, 128, 169
Kannada, 29, 95
karma, 41–42, 68
Katha Upanishads, 65–66. *See also* Upanishads
kathaka storytelling, 15
Katz, Tristan, 15
Kaushalya, 93
Kaushika, 139, 141–142
Kaushitaki Brahmana, 81
Keralolpathi, 59
Khalsa, 161
Khalsa, Harbhajan Singh, 165
Khasi, 26
King Janaka, 93
    Sulabha, 80–83
Konkani, 16
Kosala, 44
Krishna, 3
    Arjuna, 85, 91
    balakrishna, 121
    Bhagavat Purana, 115
    bhakti, 115, 119–120
    Brahmanism, appropriation, and
        sanitization, 132–133
    gender fluidity, 101
    Gita Govinda, 118–119
    Hari, 122
    historical persona, 121–123
    idol facing west, 128
    International Society for Krishna
        Consciousness (ISKCON/Hare
        Krishna), 120
    Jagannatha, 118
    Krishnayadevakiputraya, 121
    Madhava, 116
    Muslims, 120–121
    portrayal in literature, 115–124
    Radha, 111–112, 117–124, 132–133. *See
        also* Radha
    Radhakrishna, 114
    Sudama, 121

teachings on yoga, 67–68
  Vasudeva, 122
  Vishnu, 122
Krishna consciousness, 120
Krishna Dvaipayana (Vyasa), 82
Krishnamacharya, Tirumalai, 69, 104
kriya yoga, 67
Kshatriyas, 35, 37
Kundalini Yoga, 165

L

Lakshmi, 113
  Radha, 132
Lalla, 147–148
language, 11–15
  origin of word *Hindu*, 49
  term *yoga*, 64
  usage of terms *savarna*, *avarna*, and *caste*, 35
  use of word *yoga* in text, 71
  Vedic rituals, 31
languages, 24, 29, 35
  Austroasiatic, 26
  Awadhi, 130
  Dravidian, 29
  Harappan, 29
  Harappans, 95
  Indo-European, 30
  Konkani, 16
  Mahabharata and Ramayana, 44
  proto-Dravidian, 29
  regional languages and Vedic literature, 41
  Sanskrit. *See* Sanskrit
  Tamil, 29
law texts
  Dharmashastras, 54
  Manu Smritia, 94
Lévi-Strauss, Claude, 13
liberation, 70, 167. *See also* moksha
Lopamudra, 87

M

Madhava, 116
Magadhi, 35
Mahabharata, 13–14, 18, 34, 41, 44, 54–55, 68, 72, 103, 131
  composition/compilation of, 43–44, 82
  Draupadi, 101
  Ekalavya, 97
  gender fluidity, 101
  gurus, 164
  Harivamsa, 122

Radha, 114
  storytelling, 17
  Sulabha, 81–82
  translation of, 59
Mahabuddhavamsa, 17
Mahadevi, Akka, 71, 130, 138–143, 147, 149, 154, 169
  devotion to Shiva, 139–140
  life in Srishaila, 142
  nakedness, 140–141, 146
  pilgrimage to Kalyana, 140–141
  poetry, 142–143
  questioning by Basavanna, 140–142
  vachanas, 148
  wooing by Kaushika, 139
Mahalasa, 101
Mahaprabhu, Chaitanya, 119
Maharashtri, 35
Mahavira, 38
Maitreyi, 81, 87, 108
Malayalam, 29, 95
Malhotra, Anshu, 14–15
Malik Muhammad Jayasi, 60
Manava Dharmashastra. *See* Manu Smriti
Mandhata, 101
Manu Smriti (aka Manava Dharmashastra), 14, 42–43
  burning of (Manusmriti Dahan Divas), 94
  composition of, 88
  definition to whom dharma applies, 50
  ethical conduct for men, 88–89
  influence on caste, class, and gender, 106
  lack of word Hindu, 50
  pravritti dharma, 85
  preservation of class and caste, 96–97
  preservation of the varna system, 90
  prominence as law book, 94
  status of women and gender minorities, 89
  translation of, 94
Manu's codebook for good wives, 129
Manusmriti Dahan Divas, 94
Mapilla Ramayana, 59
marga, 68, 71, 124, 156. *See also* bhakti
marital rape, 105
marriage
  Akka Mahadevi, 139
  child marriage, 90
  honor killings, 105–106
  marital rape, 105
Maruts, 32
Matanga, 39

matsyanyaya, 36
meat, 33
men
    ethical conduct in Manava Dharmashastra,
        88–89
    pums prakriti, 88
    savarnas, 41–42
method, 11–15
Mill, James, 61–62
Mimamsa school of philosophy, 51
Mingus, Mia, 77
Mirabai, 128, 130
miscegeny, 92
misogyny, Bhakti movement, 130
Modi, Narendra, 5–6, 131
Mohini, 101–102
moksha, 50, 65, 68, 70, 103–104
    four purusharthas, 84
    jivanmrit, 126
    reinforcement through storytelling, 17
    Sulabha, 83–84
Muddupalani, 123
mudras, 11
Mueller, Max, 62
Mughals, 59–60
    erasure of legacy, 72
mukti, 70
multiplicities, holding, 109
Munda, 26
Muslims. *See also* Islam
    Indigeneity, 74
    Kabir. *See* Kabir
    Lal Ded, 147
    patriarchy, 154–155
    Piro. *See* Piro
    pluralism, 71–74
    polarities between Hindus and Muslims,
        61–62
    Radha and Krishna, 120–121
Mutta, 98
myths
    four levels of analysis of myth, 13
    The Myth of the Holy Cow (Jha), 33

N

nakedness, 145–146
    Akka Mahadevi, 146, 149
    Digambaras monks, 145–146
    Lal Ded, 147
Nanak, 126, 156, 159–160, 164

Nanda, Mahapadma, 36
Nappinnai, 115
nastikas and astikas, 51
Nath yogis, 72, 160
Natyashastra, 117
Navratri, celebration by yoga studios, 48
neoliberal spiritual capitalism, 4–5
    reductiveness of practice, 170
nivritti dharma, 84–86, 92, 101
nonattachment, 14, 86
nudity. *See* nakedness
Nyaya school of philosophy, 51

O

ocean metaphor for yoga, 16
Oduyanambi, 102
Omvedt, Gail, 12
Oppenheimer, Robert, 1
oral traditions, 147–148
    avarnas, 62–63
    Harivamsa, 122
    ignorance of, 147
    local or vernacular languages, 94, 96
    Mapilla Ramayana, 59
    power of, 147–148
    Ramayana, 44
    Rig Veda, 43
Orientalism (Said), 61
origin of yoga, 25
    Pashu-pati, 27–28
    Upanishads, 39
orthodoxy, x

P

Padma Purana, 116
paintings, 72
Pali, 17, 24, 35, 170
    Therigatha or Songs of the Buddhist Nuns,
        97–98
Paramatma, 70
Parvati, 113
Pashu-pati, 27–28
Patanjala yoga, 68
Patanjali, 3, 67
    convergence of Hatha yoga with Patanjali's
        yoga, 69
    definition of yoga, 66–67
    Yoga Sutras. *See* Yoga Sutras
Patanjali Ayurved, 5
Patankar, Prachi, 12, 75

pativrata, 105
patriarchy
    caste system, 86–90
    child marriage, 90
    confronting patriarchal norms, 130
    establishment of, 40
    expanding inquiries of Brahmanical
        patriarchy in yoga history, 108–109
    external modes of distinction for men,
        154–155
    gurus, 165
    in Hindu teachings, 12
    honor killings, 105–106
    marital rape, 105
    pravritti and nivritti dharma, 86
    Sanskrit as medium for Brahmanism, 94–98
    savarnas, 41–42
    sex and control, 90–94
Peero Preman (Shahryar), 157
Perumal, Cheraman, 59
Petersen, Eugenia. *See* Devi, Indra
Phule, Jyotirao, 12, 105
Phule, Savitribai, 105
Pillai, Manu, 59
Piro, 71, 151–166, 169
    bhakti for Gulabdas, 154, 157
    burial with Gulabdas, 157, 162
    Ik Sau Sath Kafian, 153–156
    meeting Gulabdas, 153–154
    self-reclamation, 152–158
pluralism, 71–74
poetry
    Akka Mahadevi, 142–143
    Bhakti poetry, 57–58, 120, 125, 157
    Bhakti poets and bridal mysticism, 138
    caste-privileged Bhakti poets, 129–131
    Ik Sau Sath Kafian (Piro), 153–156
    Kabir, 126
    Radhika Santwanam (Muddupalani), 123
    women poets, 115–116
    women's labor and drudgery, 128–129
positionality, 11–15
Prabhu, Allama, 140–141
practice, 168
prajna, 167
Prakrit, 24, 35, 170
Prakriti, 99–100
pravritti dharma, 84–86, 92, 101
    stri dharma, 90
Prithvi, 31

pums (man) prakriti, 88
Punjab, 154–155, 160–161
    Gulabdasis, 153
    Sikhism, 159
Puranas, 34, 41, 50–51, 113
    gender fluidity, 100
    gender narratives, 93
    lack of word *Hindu*, 50
    patriarchy, 102
    Radha-Lakshmi, 132
    self-referential, 43
    storytelling, 17
    yoga teacher training, 47
Puranic literature
    debates, 103
    Radha, 115
purity and pollution, 107–108
purusa, 34
    gender, 99–100
Purusa Sukhtam, 34
purusharthas, 84

Q

queer sexualities in Vedic literature, 88

R

Radha, 12, 71, 111–124, 169
    bhakti, 124–126. *See also* bhakti
    bhakti and viveka, 133–134
    Brahmanism, appropriation, and
        sanitization, 132–133
    Gatha Saptasati, 114–115
    Krishna, 111–112, 117–124, 132–133
    Muslims, 120–121
    portrayal in literature, 115–124
    Radha-rani, 120, 132
    rasa as resistance, 131–132
    Vaishnavism, 122–123
Radhakrishna, 114
Radhakrishnan, Sarvepalli, 52
Radhika Santwanam (Muddupalani), 123
Radhika. *See* Radha
Rajatarangini, 127
Rakshasas, conflicts with Devas, 37
Rama, 132
    Ramcharitmanas (Tulsidas), 130–131
Ramayana, 12, 14, 34, 41, 44, 103
    composition of, 43–44
    Mapilla Ramayana, 59
    Sita, 101

Ramayana (*continued*)
    storytelling, 17
    Valmiki Ramayana, 93
Ramcharitmanas (Tulsidas), 130–131
Ramdev, Baba, 5
rasa, 117, 125–126
    as resistance, 131–132
    sringara rasa, 131
Rashtriya Swayamsevak Sangh, 6
Razmnamah (Book of War), 59
rebirth, 41, 66
    Charvakas, 9
    karma, 42
reductiveness, 5, 8, 12
reflexivity, 43
reincarnation, 50
religion
    defined as dharma, 54
    external modes of distinction for men, 154–155
    institutionalization by British, 63
    weaponization by colonizers, 162
religious nationalism. *See* Hindutva
repair, 77
resistance, 169
    debates as, 103–106
    rasa as, 131–132
Rig Veda, 30, 41, 53
    composition of, 30
    gender fluidity, 100
    gods and goddesses, 30–31
    occupations, 36
    oral preservation, 43
    Purusa Sukhtam, 34
    references to yoga, 64
    vratyas, 39
RISE. *See* Root, Integrate, Study, and take
    Embodied Action
rishikas, 86, 108
rituals, 40, 42
    Vedic, 31–32
    wives, 42
Root, Integrate, Study, and take Embodied
    Action (RISE), 169–172
Roy, Arundathi, 79
Roy, Ram Mohan, 54

S

sacred, 18, 19
sacred resilience, 18, 19
sacrifices, Vedic pastoralists, 31–33
sahadharmini, 87

Said, Edward, 61
Sama Veda, 41
Samaj, Arya, 54
Samaj, Brahmo, 54
Samkhya school of philosophy, 51, 99
Samkhya Karika, 100
samsara, 65
samskaras, 14, 70, 107, 167
Saṃskṛtam Sanskrit, 95
sanatan dharma, 24
sangha, 39–40
Sanskrit, 7, 9, 14–15, 30, 35, 170
    as ancestral language, 106, 107
    British translation of Sanskrit texts, 62
    commentaries on texts, 69
    history of, 95
    itihasa, 16
    as medium for Brahmanism, 94–98
    Prakrit, 35
    Saṃskṛtam Sanskrit, 95
    Sulabha, 81
    Upanishads, 39
    Vedic literature, 9
    vernacularization of texts, 96
Sanskritization, 96
sant, 161–162
sanyasi ashrama, 42
sanyasis, 86
Saraswati, 31, 96–97, 113
Saraswati, Dayanand, 54
Satchidananda, 164
sat-sang, 155–156, 166
Saulubha Shakha, 81
Savarkar, Vinayak Damodar, 6, 94
savarnas, 13, 35, 41–43, 65, 84–85
scope, 11–15
seals
    Harappan society, 28–29
    Mohenjo-Daro unicorn, 23
    Pashu-pati, 27–28
section 375 of the Indian Penal Code, 105
self-awareness, 73
self-discipline, 85
self-reflection, 77
sex and control, 90–94
sexual intermingling of classes (varnasamkara),
    91–92
sexual misconduct accusations of gurus, 164–165
Shah Jahan, 60
Shahryar, 157
Shairi (Swarajbir), 157

Shaivas/Shaivites, 56–57, 126, 160
    clashes with other Bhakti factions, 127
Shaktas, 126
    clashes with other Bhakti factions, 127
Shakti, 100–101, 104
sharanas, 147
Shatapatha Brahmana, 30
Shauraseni, 35
Sheikh, Fatima, 105
Shikhandi, 101–102
Shikoh, Dara, 161
Shilavati, 101
Shiva, 51
    Akka Mahadevi, 139–141
    Bhakti movement, 115
    gender fluidity, 101
    Parvati, 113
    Shaivite. *See* Shaivas/Shaivites
    sharanas, 147
    Veerashaivas, 140
    yoga studios, 48
shlokas, 97
shruthi, 43
Shudras, 35, 131
    barring from Puranic temples, 127–128
    preservation of class and caste in Manu
        Smriti, 96–97
Shumbaka, 11
Shurpanaka, 11, 93
Shvetambara monks, 146
Sikhs/Sikhism, 159–161
    founding of, 159
    Guru Nanak, 126, 156, 159–160, 164
    identification as Hindus, 63
    outward symbols of faith, 159–160
    patriarchy, 154–155
    teachings of the Gurus, 160
    ten Gurus, 159–160
Silappadikaram, 115
Sita, 101
skin color, 34
soham, 159
Soma, 88
Songs of the Buddhist Nuns (Therigatha), 97–98
Sood, Sheena, 7
Soundararajan, Thenmozhi, ix–xii, 12, 38, 106
South Asian history, 26–27
Special Self, 67
sramanas, 9, 24, 32–33, 65, 167
Sri Guru Granth Sahib, 159
sringara rasa, 131

Srinivas, M. N., 96
storytelling, 15
    as disruptive practice, 15–18
    itihasa, 16
    kathaka, 15
    Mahabuddhavamsa, 17
    yoga history, 16–18
stri (woman) prakriti, 88
stri dharma, 90
studying history, 171
Sudama, 121
suffering (dukka), 71, 76
Sufis, 60
    al-haq, 159
    warrior asceticism, 160
Sulabha, 71, 79–83, 104, 169
    ascetic and householder (pravritti and
        nivritti dharma), 84–86
    debates as resistance, 103–106
    gender, 82–83
    gender fluidity in ancient narratives, 99–102
    Mahabharata, 81–82
    moksha, 83–84
    patriarchy as part of caste system, 86–90
    Sanskrit as ancestral language, 106–107
    Sanskrit as medium for Brahmanism, 94–98
    sex and control, 90–94
Sungha, Pushyamitra, 127
Sunya Sampadne, 141
Sutras. *See* Yoga Sutras
Sutta Nippata, 39
Svachchanda Tantra, 89
Svatmarama, 92
Swami Vivekananda, 8, 69, 122
Swarajbir, 157
syncretism, 73, 161–163

T

Take Back Yoga campaign, 8
Tamil, 29, 95
    origin, 29
Tantra, 67, 89
    Amritasiddhi, 68
    Brahmanism, 89–90
    gurus, 164
    patriarchy, 98
    Svachchanda Tantra text, 89
    yoginis, 104
tapas, 85
teacher training, xi, 47–48
Telugu, 29, 95

temples, castes, 127–128
texts, 14
    Amritasiddhi, 68
    appearance of word *yoga*, 64–65
    Bahr-al-Hayat, 60
    Bhagavad Gita. *See* Bhagavad Gita
    Bhagavat Purana, 115, 123
    British translation of, 62
    commentaries, 69
    commonalities and themes in teachings, 70
    Dattatreyayogasastra, 69
    debates, 103
    definition of yoga, 70
    denial of caste narratives, 13
    Divyadana, 127
    four levels of analysis of myth, 13
    Gatha Saptasati, 114–115
    gender bias, 102
    gender fluidity, 99–102
    Gherandasamhita, 69
    Gita Govinda, 14, 117–119, 123–124, 131
    Harivamsa, 122
    Hatha Yoga Pradipika. See Hatha Yoga Pradipika
    horse-chariot/ox-cart metaphor, 64, 66
    intertextuality, 41
    investigation into, 12
    Keralolpathi, 59
    lack of word *Hindu*, 50
    law books, 42–43, 94
    Mahabharata, 14, 54
    Manava Dharmashastra. *See* Manu Smriti
    Manu Smriti. *See* Manu Smriti
    Manu's codebook for good wives, 129
    Natyashastra, 117
    portrayals of women, 101
    preference over oral traditions, 147
    Rajatarangini, 127
    Ramayana, 14
    references to yoga, 67–69
    Samkhya Karika, 100
    Sri Guru Granth Sahib, 159
    storytelling, 17
    Sunya Sampadne, 141
    Svachchanda Tantra, 89
    Upanishads. *See* Upanishads
    Vaishnavism, 123
    Vedas. *See* Vedas
    Vedic literature and Brahmanism, 40–45
    vernacularization of Sanskrit texts, 96
Thapar, Romila, 12, 14

The Trauma of Castei (Soundararajan), 38
theism, 51–52
Therigatha or Songs of the Buddhist Nuns, 97–98
timiti, 18
transformation, 168
transnational yoga, 25
trittiya prakriti, 88
Tulsidas, 130

U

understanding, 73
Universal Consciousness, 159
untouchability, 38
    Chandala, 39
upanayam, 11
Upanishads, 8, 14, 25, 39, 41, 55, 163
    Atma, 99, 109
    Atma and Brahman, 81
    Chandogya Upanishad, 121
    composition of, 39
    consciousness and matter, 70
    debates as resistance, 103
    Gargi, 81
    gender fluidity, 82, 99
    gurus, 164
    horse-chariot/ox-cart metaphor, 64, 66
    Krishna, 121–122
    lack of word *Hindu*, 50
    Maitreyi, 81
    mention of yoga, 65–66
    preference over oral traditions, 147
    Radha, 114
    Sankaracharya's commentaries, 69
    self-referential, 43
    storytelling, 17
    translation of, 60, 62, 161
    yoga, 39, 68, 70
    yoga teacher training, 47
Urdu, 159
Ushas, 31
Uttar Pradesh, 44

V

vachanas, 147–148
vairagya, 14, 86
Vaisheshika school of philosophy, 51
Vaishnavas/Vaishnavism/Vaishnavites, 56–57,
    122–123, 126, 160
    clashes with other Bhakti factions, 127
    Radha-rani, 132
Vaishyas, 35

Vak, 31, 100
vakhs, 147–148
Valmiki Ramayana, archetypes, 93
vanaprastha ashrama, 86
Vanita, Ruth, 14, 81, 103
Vardhamana Mahavira, 65
varna-jaatis, 12
varnas, 34–37, 50
    Sulabha, 83
varnasamkara, 91–92
Varuna, 30, 97
Vaselasutta, 39
Vasudeva, 122
Vedanta, Din-Ilahi, 161
Vedanta school of philosophy, 51
Vedas, 9, 14, 20, 24, 31, 33, 40–45, 50, 55–56, 163
    archetypes in Vedic Brahmanism, 93
    astikas, 51
    Atharva Veda, 32
    British translation of, 62
    composition of, 95
    diverse gender identities and queer
        sexualities, 88
    gods, 97
    gurus, 164
    homosexual relationships among deities, 88
    Indigeneity, 74
    influence of Indigenous cultures, 37
    intertextuality, 41
    Krishna, 121
    lack of word *Hindu*, 50
    law texts, 42–43
    primary composers, 27
    Radha, 114
    Rig Veda, 30, 34, 36, 39, 41, 43, 53, 64, 100
    rishikas, 86
    Sanskrit, 9
    savarnas, 41–42
    self-referential, 43
    Vishnu, 122
    women, 87
Vedic Age, 35
Vedic astrology, 88
Vedic Brahmanism, 9, 65
Vedic pastoralists, 30–33
Vedic Samhitas, 41
Veerashaivas, 140
vegetarianism, 32–33, 108
vernacularization of Sanskrit texts, 96
Vijjakka, 97
village deities (grama devatas), 124

violence
    Bhakti factions, 127
    honor killings, 105–106
    marital rape, 105
    pravritti dharma, 85
    prior to Islamic rulers, 127
Vishnu, 11, 51
    avatars of, 122–123
    Balarama, 122
    Bhakti movement, 115
    Krishna, 122
    Puranas, 17
    Vaishnavism, 122–123
    Vaishnavite, 56–57
    yoga studios, 48
Vithoba, 129, 130, 132
viveka, 133–134
Vivekananda, Swami, 8, 63, 69, 122
vratyas, 39
Vrijis, 38
vyakta, 82–83
Vyasa, 82

W

white supremacy, 170
women
    Akka Mahadevi. *See* Mahadevi, Akka
    archetypes in Valmiki Ramayana, 93–94
    authors, 97
    Bhimbekta cave paintings, 87
    Brahmin women's sexuality, 90–91
    bridal mysticism, 138–139
    Buddha, 97–98
    Dasa women of conquered tribes, 91
    feminist resistance to caste, 105
    hatha yoga, 92–93, 102
    inaccessibility of classical Sanskrit, 97
    Manu's codebook for good wives, 129
    Piro. *See* Piro
    poems by, 115–116
    poetry about labor and drudgery, 128–129
    portrayals in texts, 101
    pravritti and nivritti dharma, 85–86
    savarna, 41
    savarnas, 42
    status in Manava Dharmashastra, 89
    stri prakriti, 88
    tantra, 67
    Vedas, 87
    yoga, 104
    yoginis, 81–82, 86, 93, 104

Y

Yadavas, 38
yajnas, 31
Yajur Veda, 41
yoga
  appropriation and appreciation of, 74, 75, 76, 77
  bhakti marga, 68, 71, 124, 156. *See also* bhakti
  bhakti yoga, 124, 134
  Chaturanga, 48
  cocreating welcoming yoga spaces, 170
  definition of, 64–70
  embedded within social context of times, 3–4
  embodiment practices, 148–149
  gurus, 163–166
  hatha yoga, 68
  history. *See* yoga history
  interrogate narratives around purity and pollution, 107–108
  kriya yoga, 67
  mainstream exclusion of histories of religions, colonialism, and castes, 63
  ocean metaphor, 16
  origin. *See* origin of yoga
  overlap with "religion", 124
  purity and pollution, 108
  purpose of, 70–71
  Sanskrit as ancestral language, 106–107
  synergies between Islam and yoga, 72
  term *yoga*, 64
  transnational, 25
  Upanishads, 39, 70
  use of word *yoga* in text, 71
  weaponization in nationalist movements and ideologies, 169

yoga history, 2–5
  convergence of Hatha yoga and Patanjali's yoga, 69
  conveyed through storytelling, 16–18
  early text references to yoga, 67–69
  expanding inquiries of Brahmanical patriarchy, 108–109
  heterodoxy, 9–10
  Hindutva, 5–11
  neoliberal spiritual capitalism, 4–5
  reexamining, 4–5
  resistance against oppression, 3–4
  women, 104
Yoga school of philosophy, 51
yoga studios, deity idols and festival celebrations, 48
Yoga Sutras, 3, 8, 25
  definition of yoga, 66–67, 70
  expanding inquiries of Brahmanical patriarchy, 109
  gender fluidity, 99
  mention of yoga, 66
  preference over oral traditions, 147
  references to asana, 68
  Vyasa's commentary, 69
  yoga teacher training, 47
yoga teacher training, xi, 47–48
yoga, and Hindu, 47–53
  definition of yoga, 64–70
  dharma, 53–56
  genesis of "Hindu" label, 56–64
  teacher training and yoga studios, 47–48
Yogi Bhajan, 164–165
yoginis, 81–82, 86, 93, 104
Yuvanashva, 101

Acknowledgments

This book is an offering of love to yoga practitioners who are unafraid to ask difficult questions of themselves, of yoga, and of me. Writing is a lonely process, and you were the inspiration for the work. I sincerely hope you take it forward, queer the yoga spaces, and make them better.

There are so many people who have made this possible for me. I start with the one who knows me the most, Yatin, the one whom I lean on for the best chai in town, grammar checks, silly humor, and a steadfastness that holds me without stifling.

Gratitude for Thenmozhi Soundararajan for writing the powerful foreword. Thenmozhi's support and our conversations about yoga, Hindutva, and caste were integral in the development of this work.

I have learned much from the work of Prachi Patankar, who continues to blaze untrodden paths toward an anticaste and antifascist future. Thank you, Prachi, for your unwavering voice and friendship.

A heartfelt thank you to my academic advisor and professor at the California Institute of Integral Studies, Dr. Alka Arora, who read through every line of the manuscript and gave me encouragement as well as critical feedback. The book is better because of her, and all errors are mine alone.

Thank you to Shayna Keyles, editor, for your sharp input, immense patience, and friendly disposition that made it easy to ask basic questions about the publishing process.

I never thought writing a book was a remote possibility for me until Jivana Heyman mentioned it to me when we were working together in the Accessible Yoga Association. Many may say it, but he really meant it as he followed up with next steps on how I should go about it. Thank you, Jivana, for your friendship and mentorship, reading the early draft of the manuscript, and our thousands of texts back and forth on all things yoga and life.

To my friend Tristan Katz, who read the book proposal and cheered me every step of the way. Someday soon I hope to do the same for you and read your book. The world will be better for it.

Thank you to Michelle Cassandra Johnson, whose book *Skill in Action* articulated how yoga can be a radical practice of personal and collective transformation. I read it in the first year of the pandemic, and it lit up my path.

To my siblings, Leena and Harish, I know you will have my back, as I will yours. Thank you to my dad, Lakshman, who taught me to ask questions and read all kinds of books; and to my mom, Meera, who said a prayer is a conversation with the sacred.

And my beloved children, Ishan and Ayana, I love you with every fiber of my being. Being your mom is the greatest gift.

Five percent of this book's sales will be donated to the Miss Major Alexander L. Lee TGIJP Black Trans Cultural Center. The TGI Justice Project (TGIJP) is a group of transgender, gender-variant, and intersex (TGI) people inside and outside of prisons, jails, and detention centers creating a united family in the struggle for survival and freedom. We work to forge a culture of resistance and resilience to strengthen us for the fight against human rights abuses, imprisonment, police violence, racism, poverty, and societal pressures for Black and Black/Brown TGI people. We seek to create a world rooted in self-determination, freedom of expression, and gender justice. Please find us at https://tgijp.org/.

About the Author

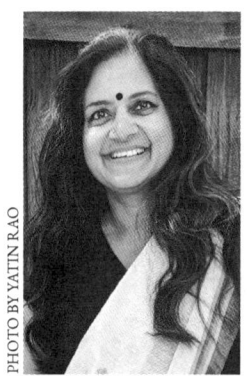

Anjali Rao is an enthusiastic questioner and a fervent seeker of truths. She is a yoga educator and practitioner who offers insight into the stories and histories obscured by heteropatriarchy and colonization. Her work deconstructs the dynamics of power in yoga, integrating art, philosophy, and history. Anjali is an Indian American immigrant and a cancer survivor, and she is on the faculty of many national and international programs for continuing education in yoga. She is the host of *The Love of Yoga* podcast, where she shares thought-provoking conversations with yoga scholars and activists on the front lines of liberatory movements. Anjali is currently pursuing a doctorate in philosophy and religion in a transdisciplinary program at the intersections of feminist, religious, philosophical, and Indigenous thought. She is partial to dark chocolate, old trees, and cheeky puppies.

About North Atlantic Books

North Atlantic Books (NAB) is an independent, nonprofit publisher committed to a bold exploration of the relationships between mind, body, spirit, and nature. Founded in 1974, NAB aims to nurture a holistic view of the arts, sciences, humanities, and healing. To make a donation or to learn more about our books, authors, events, and newsletter, please visit www.north atlanticbooks.com.

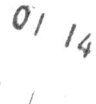